THE EMPOWERED MIND DIET EQUATION

Get To The Best Version Of Yourself
Via Diet & Mind

By
Rika Mansingh, RD

The Empowered Mind Diet Equation
Copyright © 2018 by Rika Mansingh

All rights reserved. No part of this publication may be
reproduced, distributed, or transmitted in any form or
by any means, including photocopying, recording, or
other electronic or mechanical methods, without the prior
written permission of the author, except in the case of brief
quotations embodied in critical reviews and certain other
non-commercial uses permitted by copyright law.

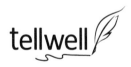

Tellwell Talent
www.tellwell.ca

ISBN
978-0-2288-0949-4 (Hardcover)
978-0-2288-0758-2 (Paperback)
978-0-2288-0759-9 (eBook)

TABLE OF CONTENTS

PREFACE

If you're picking up this book, I take it you have been on your own challenging journey, and it has brought you to this point — you're seeking something more. You want more energy and vitality and want to conquer your brain, maximizing its use for optimal health and well-being. Congratulations on getting here, and be grateful for reaching this point in your life where you are eager to improve your state of mind and become the best version of yourself — the place where you once may have been or a place you are striving to reach.

I have been on my journey, which I am grateful for — a journey of the mind and, like you, I have searched for resources to elevate me. I wanted to maximize my energy and empower my brain and, for me, learning has been key. Knowledge has been power. I wanted to rise up and become the best version of myself, with the least amount of effort, of course. Just give me the science and tools, and it would have the credibility to make me diligent enough to comply. Life is busy and chaotic, and with limited time, we all want to learn in the quickest way possible and achieve a positive ripple effect in our lives. I would hear audios on high speeds to gain concentrated, concise, yet impactful knowledge, and that is what I intend to provide you in this book. I have been through the scientific literature and have broken it down to present material in a way that is easy to understand and practical to follow. There is a lot of information to go through, but my aim is simplicity — you will go through the book quickly and still feel moved and empowered and, most of all, by the end of it and after adopting the principles, you will have a clear mind, better mood, enhanced memory, uninterrupted and replenished sleep, revitalized energy and, most importantly, happiness because of it all.

So, guess what, after decades of believing the brain is static and cannot change, this is no longer true. New findings in the field of neuroscience and with neurogenesis and neuroplasticity, neuroscientists have now realized that the brain can change. We can actually repair damaged brain cells or even rewire our brain to change thought patterns and behaviours.

This book will equip you with the knowledge to do this, with an emphasis on diet, and it is now what I have come to call *The Empowered Mind Diet Equation*. Healthy thoughts + healthy food = a healthy mind. A healthy mind + healthy thoughts = healthy behaviours that lead to happiness.

And my mind diet for wellness algorithm:

IF you change your thoughts and change your diet, THEN you change your mind to become the best and most authentic version of yourself. Eat well, think well, feel well, and rewire your brain. Enjoy the read!

INTRODUCTION: MY JOURNEY, MY MIND

So, How Did I Get Here?

Earlier on in my journey and while growing up, I heard the saying, "life is like a roller coaster ride." I knew there would be ups and downs, with good days and bad days, and I knew that when there are bad days, "this too shall pass," and it wouldn't be long before I picked up again, as long as I stayed on the track.

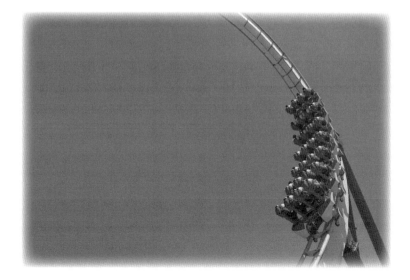

My roller coaster ride during childhood and into adulthood was magnificent. I had been blessed to grow up in a wonderful loving family, my pillar of strength, loving and inspiring dad, my strong, caring and motivational mum, my creative and thoughtful brother, and an energetic extended family who created a lively atmosphere with an abundance of music, dancing and singing. I qualified as a registered dietitian in South Africa in 2002. While in South Africa, I worked as a clinical dietitian and consultant dietitian in private practice. I also did media work for the newspaper, radio, and satellite TV. My roller coaster had soaring heights and breathtaking precious moments, which I am very grateful for, to this day.

After getting married, I moved to Canada. So young, excited and enthusiastic to move to a country I had never visited before. Experiencing snow for the very first time was beautiful. Learning how to drive on the other side of the road was an exciting challenge. Day by day, I was amazed at the warm friendliness of Canadian people despite the cold weather.

I continued on my journey, still on my roller coaster ride, as life continued, and then suddenly I find myself viciously jolted on my roller coaster track.

Here I am sitting in my roller coaster cart, and it is no longer going up into the clear blue sky but instead crashing through a series of downward spirals. I was going through a divorce. For those of you who have been through a divorce or any difficult situation or similar circumstance, you would agree when I say, it is definitely not easy.

There were challenging emotions day by day, and l had to learn how to master them and control them before they controlled me. The key is to stay on track. We are emotional human beings and often emotions, if not transformed from negative to positive, can get the better of us and, in doing so, our energy levels are affected, sleep is disturbed, our appetite changes — we lose our appetite completely, or for others, crave huge amounts of unhealthy food for comfort.

I realized that I had to rely on my own mind to carry me through this difficult time. My mind had to be strong. How do we pick our minds up to find our way again? How do we stay on our roller coaster track of life without being derailed when difficult situations arise?

While on my roller coaster, I once met a girl in a restaurant who had an interesting tattoo on her hand. I had always been so curious about people and their journeys and seek every opportunity to learn from them. We can learn from anyone we meet. We can learn from anything at all, actually, from as small as a brave mosquito to as large as a powerful, fearless lion. I curiously asked this girl with the bow and arrow tattoo, "What made you get a bow and arrow tattoo?" Her reply was something I will always remember, a response that had made a massive impact on my mind and how I moved forward afterward, by literally moving backward. She said, "The bow and arrow — sometimes we have to take a few steps back before we can move full steam ahead." A simple conversation shot an arrow to my mind and directed it to focus on being grateful.

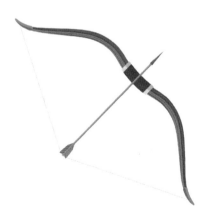

We have all heard the old adage, "What doesn't kill you makes you stronger." It truly does. Our setbacks make us stronger; they are blessings in disguise. We just have to find the blessings and be grateful. In time, I realized my biggest enemy was stagnation. Those moments, that phase, of feeling like a victim, which is natural at the beginning of difficult situations, had to pass. Many books and audiobooks later, I realized that there is nothing more disempowering than assuming a victim-like role in an unpleasant situation. I had realized that no matter what circumstances the universe sends our way — the way we handle it — it all boils down to two words: OUR CHOICE. We decide how we allow situations to affect us. We give the situation the power to control us, or we take control and become empowered by it. I chose the latter.

I had made a decision to *try* to be strong and independent here in Canada while my family was back in South Africa. After all the studying I had completed to be here, I wanted to continue to follow my passion and become a successful dietitian in Canada. I had a gut feeling that my purpose in life was to help people through food and nutrition, and I was determined to follow it.

I wanted to take control and feel empowered. I did countless classes of Zumba, yoga and other gym routines. We all know how important exercise is, for general fitness, mental health, and well-being. The natural high from endorphin release after exercise is both extremely refreshing, addictive and does wonders for sleep. But what happens when we don't have the energy to exercise after a long day at work or in the morning after insufficient sleep while going through a challenging situation? What happens if our minds can't take us to where we want to go? That's the missing step. It all starts with our minds and being able to direct it to where we want to take it — to achieve and conquer our goals.

We know about having faith and belief. Believing and having faith in a higher power, or that something good is still about to happen, requires a strong mindset. The power of positive thinking. How do we have faith and belief and think positive thoughts with a lack of energy to do exercise, a lack of sleep, a lack of focus and concentration? Positive thinking works better with a strategy. That's how we really optimize the effects of positive thinking — combining it with a strategy.

My strategy was to focus on the mind. Focusing on the mind would lead to better thinking — more faith, belief, the enhanced ability to transform negative emotions into positive emotions, improved mood, concentration, better memory — our minds are our most important asset. With a strong, solid mind, we can truly overcome any difficult situation or achieve any goal.

Being a dietitian, I targeted my focus on nutrition for the mind. I decided to explore this area of nutrition further and found that by incorporating certain foods and other nutrition components to my diet, I had experienced the benefits of improved mood, higher energy levels, better concentration, and uninterrupted sleep. Whether I did exercise or not, I still felt amazing.

Happiness comes from within. Happiness is a state of mind and a choice — a choice that only a healthy mind can make. After teaching classes and running workshops about healthy eating for diabetes, heart-healthy eating, and healthy eating to manage weight, I found that the key to happiness in abundance was helping people. It brought me tremendous joy to have a positive impact on patients' lives and make a difference to their well-being.

After learning about neurogenesis, neuroplasticity, eating healthily for the brain, trying it out for myself and sharing this with my patients — I found myself and many of my patients, feeling happy, energized and, most of all, resilient. I see food as information for the brain. If we are mindful of what we eat and how it makes us feel, this constant association generates healthy behaviours ensuring we feel at our best.

Eat well to feel well. I am grateful for my journey, and I wanted to share what I have learned, linking the mind and diet to wellness.

I obtained my full registration with the College of Dietitians BC and became a member of Dietitians of Canada. Since doing so, I am currently working in long-term care and doing private practice in the Abbotsford area, have conducted nutrition workshops in Langley, Abbotsford, and Chilliwack and led nutrition store tours at numerous locations in the Fraser Valley. I am also currently involved in media work, write nutrition-related articles for newspapers and magazines and engaged in nutrition events linking diet and the mind.

I decided to write the *Empowered Mind Diet Equation* to help all those people who have been through or going through difficult circumstances in their life or those who just need a lifestyle boost and to assist them to improve their mood, concentration, and sleep by focusing on nutrition and empowering the mind. Eating well for the mind leads to feeling well, which in turn leads to sleeping well and more energy to exercise well. Feeding the brain is crucial for good mental health and general well-being.

CHAPTER 1

"The Only Thing That is Constant is Change." (Heraclitus)

For decades, scientists believed that we are born with a fixed number of brain cells (called neurons). If we damage them with unhealthy lifestyle choices as we age, we might not repair them or make new brain cells. It is empowering to know that this is no longer true. Research in the field of neuroscience has shown that we can actually produce new neurons at any age.

Neurogenesis is the production of new neurons and takes place in the hippocampus of the brain. The hippocampus is the area of the brain required for learning and memory. There are over 100 billion neurons in the brain, and these neurons communicate with each other through connections called synapses. These form the neuronal network of the brain.

Neuroplasticity is the brain's ability to restructure and repair itself. The brain is far more flexible than previously thought and constantly changing — it can be moulded and altered to become smarter and more creative, more resilient, and adaptable to change, have better memory while preventing cognitive decline, and have increased longevity.

So, did you ever feel stuck in a brain-foggy state? Memory was hazy, you were tired and lethargic? Needed a boost of energy to seize the day but just couldn't get your mind to elevate you? We have all been there at some point, and sometimes we can unknowingly and easily dwell in the negativity bias of the brain.

What is the negativity bias of the brain?

It's the brains tendency to focus on negative thoughts as a means of survival, usually stemming from fear. If we don't defeat the negativity bias of the brain, we could stay in this counterproductive mindset not realizing that these thought patterns are actually prolonging these cloudy feelings and altering the neuronal network of the brain, wiring it to stay negative.

These negative mindsets will have long-term effects such as low mood, feelings of hopelessness or helplessness, or you may even feel as though you're living in a state of constant alarm. It is OK to feel those emotions — they are meant to move us and teach us about ourselves. It is important to realize it, process it, learn the lessons and be mindful to observe these emotions and let them pass through or transform them to positive emotions.

Conquer fear by nurturing courage and confidence. If we don't, these negative feelings, which generate electrical impulses, actually alter brainwaves, and over time this could affect not only your mood but your personality and behaviour as well the structure of the brain. The good news is we can feel better by boosting our neurons to change our brain.

Neurogenesis occurs mainly by increasing a protein called **Brain-Derived Neurotrophic Factor (BDNF),** which preserves the neurons you have, keeping them healthy, and promoting the growth of new neurons from brain stem cells.

So, what does all this neuroscientific jargon mean? Basically, you are not stuck with the brain you have — you can alter it and there is no better time than NOW. Psychiatrist and brain disorder specialist Daniel Amen, founder of the Amen clinics, studied over 85,000 brain scans and is a firm believer that we can change our brain.

Here's how to rewire your brain, boost BDNF, and increase neurogenesis.

1) **Get thirsty for knowledge – Learn, learn, learn and challenge your brain**

I know you may be thinking, "Learn what? I don't have time? I'm done with school? Sounds so boring and time-consuming!" It's not at all that. When you make an association with learning something new each day and how it makes you feel afterwards (happier, more alert, focused and empowered), you will NEVER want to stop learning. Be mindful of learning and the effects.

Learning is known to build up cognitive reserve, an important concept in brain health. The more we build our cognitive reserve, the better our brains will function, even if exposed to stress, surgery, and toxins such as alcohol or toxins from the environment.

It's like our brains bounce back into action, more resilient, helping us cope better, equipping us to move forward. The more you challenge your brain by learning, the more you build and sustain cognitive reserve, making the brain more resilient to degenerative brain changes associated with dementia and other brain diseases.

So, learn anything on ANY subject that interests you. It could be a new language or a new skill. Learn from audiobooks or podcasts, you name it — teach your brain new things and your brain will be grateful and give you the gift of mind power to continue to learn even more, with better memory and sharper focus. The brain is fascinating that way and can do so much. Make the most of it.

Learning also reduces cognitive decline by building new neurons in the brain and restructures neuronal networks making them flexible and adaptable to change. Approach every day as a learning day.

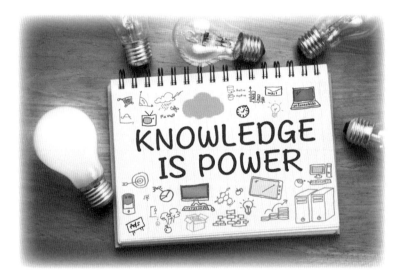

2) Eat brain wise

Diet will be explored in detail in later chapters, but for now, digest these brain-boosting points:

✓   Omega-3 for a brainy me

Omega-3 essential fatty acids such as EPA (eicosapentanoic acid) and DHA (docosahexanoic acid) promote neurogenesis and enhance brain function. Omega-3s reduce stress hormones such as cortisol and are known to be beneficial for many mental health problems. Research indicates its positive effects in reducing inflammation, improving anxiety and depression. Omega-3s also boost brain performance and can help prevent cognitive decline.

Omega-3 EPA and DHA are found in fish such as salmon, herring, sardines, mackerel, and halibut. A supplement of 1000 mg/day containing a combination of EPA and DHA would be ideal especially if not consuming fish 2–3x/wk. Algae is the vegetarian source of omega-3s available in supplement form.

✓ Come on in, curcumin

Curcumin a compound found in turmeric is known to increase BDNF and boost neurogenesis. It is also a powerful antioxidant and known for its anti-inflammatory properties as well as its role in improving symptoms of depression and Alzheimer's disease. Tumeric is highly water soluble, so you would want to take about 500 mg twice a day for it to be effective in your body over a longer time.

✓ Cheers to green tea

The brains cup of tea is most definitely green tea as it is known to contain a compound called Epigallocatechin-3-gallate (EGCG), which increases neurogenesis and regenerates damaged neurons. The greener the tea the more potent it is. Try organic ceremonial matcha tea (more about its magic later).

✓ Bring on the berries

Blueberries and cranberries, in particular, are known to have protective effects on the brain and studies have shown that blueberries can reduce your risk of Alzheimer's disease. They contain powerful antioxidants called anthocyanins (which cross the blood-brain barrier of the brain) and phytochemicals that protect neurons from oxidative damage.

If you're choosing a fruit to maximize your learning, improve thinking, and boost your memory, you might as well choose blueberries — the best fruit for the brain. More about these *berry*licious berries later.

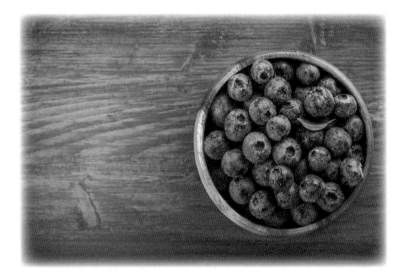

✓ Make reservations for resveratrol

Resveratrol is a natural polyphenol derived from grapes and is known to boost blood flow to the brain, increase neurogenesis, enhance brain function and memory.

Many diets recommend a glass of red wine a day as it contains resveratrol but let this resonate — There is only 4.9 mg of resveratrol per 5 oz (150 ml) glass of red wine when we need 100 mg two times per day, so best to go with a supplement as more than 1–2 glasses of wine, like all other forms of alcohol, will have the opposite effect on your brain and damage brain cells.

✓ Cut your calories

Excess calories lead to weight gain and studies have shown that the more overweight a person is, the smaller the hippocampus (memory centre of the brain). Caloric restriction can protect the brain. Being careful about the calories, reducing them by just 30 % daily, can improve memory and cognition by increasing the brain-loving BDNF mentioned earlier. Give your brain the neuroprotection it deserves and it will feed you with better cognition.

Research also indicates that intermittent fasting increases BDNF and promotes the growth of new neurons. An intermittent fast means skipping a day of eating and doing fluids and herbal teas. If that's too extreme maybe try to leave a gap of 10–12 hours between supper on one night and the next time you devour. Not so fast, though — always remember to consult your physician or health professional prior to embarking on intermittent fasting.

Consuming foods that cause inflammation, having a diet high in sugar, deficiencies in vitamin A and B, consuming fried foods and drinking alcohol in excess, all decrease neurogenesis (more about all this coming up later).

3) Movement is life

One of the best ways to boost BDNF and increase brain cells in the hippocampus of the brain is exercise and, more specifically, aerobic exercises such as running, cycling, and swimming. Exercise increases blood flow to the brain, changes brain plasticity, and improves learning and memory.

If you want your brain to function at its best, you have to keep on moving and it will have a profound influence on how you feel. Exercise also releases feel-good chemicals such as endorphins, which will boost your mood and help improve sleep.

According to Harvard research, just 2.5 hours of aerobic exercise per week is known to increase white and grey matter in the brain, which prevents age-related cognitive loss and counteracts brain volume decline even in people who already have dementia.

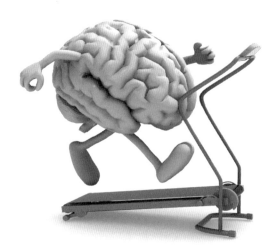

Exercise also prevents brain shrinkage in the hippocampus and prefrontal cortex of the brain and enhances cognitive functioning, reduces impulsivity and promotes better decision-making. Making the wise decision to add on resistance training 2 x 30 minutes per week will have a positive impact on your memory and attention span and also prevent brain aging and shrinkage.

Harvard research also indicates that mind-body exercises such as Yoga and Tai chi also benefit the brain by inducing physical and mental relaxation, improving one's ability to acquire, retain and retrieve information as well as boost memory.

Be mindful of your movements daily. If you do an hour of exercise in the morning but spend over 14 hours watching TV or hardly moving at all, it would defeat the purpose as prolonged hours of TV are known to decrease neurogenesis.

Move it or lose it! Make time — schedule your exercise program into your diary, the same way you would schedule an appointment with your physician or dentist. With consistent exercise routines, you can change your neuronal network, wiring it to elevate you, giving you a healthier brain and the vitality you deserve. When your brain feels healthy you will feel happier and more motivated to persevere to reach your goals.

4) Meditation, the most natural medication

Almost every time the word meditation comes up in a conversation, people often state that they don't have time or are too restless and that their minds are too busy to meditate. There are often perceptions that are conveyed, conjuring up images in one's mind that, in order to meditate, one has to sit cross-legged in a quiet corner staring into space, silencing the mind for hours. Stop the clock! Meditation doesn't have to be that way. The main idea, which I am sure we can all do for just 15–20 minutes a day, is to be present in the moment, be mindful of your breath, inhaling deeply and exhaling slowly, letting go of judgment and negativity, allowing thoughts and feelings to gently pass through. This can be done while walking or exercising, cooking, showering or even sitting at your desk. Just stop. Breathe. Be mindful of your breath.

And here's why — Numerous studies indicate that meditation increases BDNF to grow new brain cells, it increases the hippocampal grey matter in the brain and improves memory, focus and sleep.

Meditation is also known to shrink the amygdala, the fear centre of the brain. This is a mind game changer because if you think of it, FEAR is the route of all negative emotions. If you reduce fear through meditation, you will ease off focusing on the negative emotions and will move from a state of constant alarm to a much preferred, state of calm. Inhale positivity, exhale negativity and reap the, I like to say, "brainefits".

Stress and depression decrease neurogenesis. Oxidative stress from the environment such as air pollution, smoking, and pesticides also decrease neurogenesis.

5) Neuronal "leisure" and fun in the sun

Everything in life is all about balance. I like to view our neurons as little buddies in our brains. They love communicating with each other and their connections work best after having fun in the sun and doing pleasurable activities.

I call it neuronal "leisure". Our neurons need leisure time and exciting activities to fire away and spark with each other the way they should. Not only do new brain cells form but also, the connections between brain cells strengthen and rewire the structure of the brain.

Our fellow neuron buddies want to travel and explore, dance, write, read, paint, cook up a creative storm or listen to music. Spending a little time in the sun makes your body produce more vitamin D, which also increases BDNF. Gardening is great. Spending time around nature is naturally what the brain wants.

6) Healthy relationships and social connections

There is an excellent quote by a well-known, motivational speaker Jim Rohn who stated, "You are the average of the five people you spend the most time with." So, choose wisely. Healthy, positive relationships and good social connections will send out positive vibrations to your neurons and give you blissful feelings of joy, love, and excitement and, in doing so, will increase brain cells.

Always evaluate how you feel in your relationships and after social interactions — if you're feeling heavy and drained it's best to re-evaluate these connections as, in the long term, they will affect the neuronal networks in your brain. Try getting into a habit of asking yourself, "Does this interaction or connection enhance my life positively or take away from it?" Unhealthy relationships decrease neurogenesis. You want to feel energized and refreshed after social interactions and not tired or exhausted with loads of uneasiness.

A love relationship is ideal, but you don't have to be in a relationship to be happy. What's healthy is that you communicate with people, make healthy connections and surround yourself with positive energy. And hey, even if you're living on your own — audiobooks and podcasts are fantastic ways to surround yourself with the powerful company of five authors, for example. It's great! Again that quote, "You are the average of the five people you spend the most time with." Definitely a quote to high five to.

Sleep – the brain cleanser

It is a no-brainer that we need to sleep well to make the most of our days but did you know that while we sleep our brain actually gets, you could say, "cleansed" by a clear, colourless fluid called cerebrospinal fluid. Cerebrospinal fluid, found in the brain and spinal cord, flushes out the brain and helps remove beta-amyloid protein buildup. Beta-amyloid protein plaques cause memory decline as seen in Alzheimer's disease.

Harvard research shows that for every hour of awake time during the day you need a full half an hour of sleep time to process the new information you learned. Usually, 7–9 hours is essential.

Ever noticed that after poor or interrupted sleep that you toss and turn your way into engulfing more food the next day, especially craving sugar and other high carbohydrate foods and, in doing so, tend to pack on the pounds?

Here's one of the reasons:

Studies have found that lack of sleep alters useful hormones in our body, grelin, which regulates hunger and leptin, the hormone that regulates our feeling of fullness after eating. Grelin increases after sleeping poorly, making us have cravings the next day and leptin decreases, which means we don't really feel a sense of fullness after eating. Bottom line — if you're not sleeping well, you're more likely to overeat and gain weight. This will affect your mood and sleep patterns further. We need to break this cycle. Lack of sleep decreases neurogenesis, alters memory, concentration, mood, reasoning, decision-making and processing speeds.

If we are mindful of incorporating ways to boost neurogenesis discussed above, sleep, mood and cognitive functioning will improve. According to Harvard research, six months is enough to produce functional changes in the brain.

The other promising and empowering concept I would love to quickly introduce to you is epigenetics. I often see patients who tell me that they have a family history of health problems, it could be anything from diabetes, Alzheimer's disease, obesity, you name it and they would state its genetic and out of their control so any intervention would be pointless as they are inevitably going to fall prey to these conditions. Guess what? Good news again. We can move from victim to victorious through a new science called epigenetics, where researchers now realize that yes we can't change our genes but WE CAN change the way our genes are expressed and this can help prevent many hereditary health problems.

So, very simply, through epigenetics, we realize that DNA is no longer everything. With diet and healthy lifestyle changes we can actually produce chemical tags, which attach *above* our DNA, hence the term *epi*genetics. These chemical tags or epigenetic tags can cause DNA to open up or close down either turning off the genes we don't want (the genes that cause inflammation and generate free radicals) or turning on the protective genes we want (like genes that code for BDNF discussed earlier in neurogenesis).

Visualize a spiral spring as being our DNA, which contains our genes — when the spring is stretched apart, our DNA opens up exposing genes to be turned on. When the spring is condensed closer together, our genes are turned off. The chemical tags that attach to DNA give instructions to DNA and affect how the cells read underlying genes encoded in DNA.

Bottom line, we can take the lead and have a positive impact on our genes by making healthy lifestyle choices. According to Gary L. Graham from Hawthorne University, less than 2 % of human disease is a result of genetic destiny and over 95 % is epigenetically determined. Knowing this is empowering for sure. Food choices, stress, sleep, exercise, and healthy relationships can alter our gene expression and affect our health and longevity, so let's take control and be mindful on our path to wellness.

CHAPTER 2

Empower Your Thoughts, Empower Your Mind.

The mind can be our biggest barrier to change or best catalyst to bring about change, depending on how we wire it. I see many patients who strive to reach their goals to lose weight, control blood sugars, stop cravings, change disordered eating patterns — you name it. Making healthier food choices for the brain is crucial to achieving goals because food is information for the brain; it affects how we feel and places us in a healthier state of mind. But "eat this" first — achieving dietary goals or conquering any other goals, all starts with the mind. Only an empowered, positive mind can help us reach our goals, so let's get empowered!

In Chapter 1, I briefly covered the negativity bias of the brain and how crucial it is for us to defeat this bias, more so because negative thoughts create electrical impulses, which can alter the structure of the brain wiring it to be more negative.

Negative thoughts, if not nipped in the bud, can lead to a downward spiral of negative feelings, fuelling a series of negative behaviours. We can easily get caught up in a vicious cycle of negative behaviour, which can escalate to produce more negative feelings and further negative thought patterns. It is basically a negative feedback loop beginning at the thought level.

Continuation of this cycle can have harmful effects on the body, both physically and mentally. Positive thoughts generate positive feelings and lead to healthier behaviours. So, break the negative cycle. "Go cycling" with positive.

There's a quote by Buddha that states, "Rule the mind or it will rule you." How true! The mind, in essence, controls the brain. To control the brain, we must control the mind, and this begins with controlling our thoughts. How do we do this? By being mindfully aware of them.

Our thoughts can be harmful or helpful. They can elevate us, energize us, make us more productive and creative, or they could cripple us, drain us, sabotage our minds, and throw us off track completely. Our thoughts basically create and shape our reality.

If we believe these thoughts, we will actually behave in a way that makes it a reality. Also, we truly become what we believe about ourselves, so best to not give in to self-defeating thought patterns, if we want to bring about positive changes in our lives.

When we sprout a negative thought, we should really take a step back, challenge these thoughts and question them before letting them pass through or transforming them to positive. Just because we think negative thoughts almost automatically, it doesn't always mean they are true. So, the next time you're on the verge of collapsing into a negative thought pattern, try asking yourself, is this thought really true? How does believing this thought make me feel? Is it a fact or something streaming through from the subconscious mind as an altered perception? Is this belief empowering? If not, why am I believing it and giving this irrational thought the power to dampen the way I feel?

If you "think of it", our thoughts are just perceptions stemming from our subconscious mind, which has been conditioned or programmed to think in a certain way for decades. If we change the way we perceive our thoughts, we can change the way we feel and adopt healthier mindsets and behaviours.

Why focus on the negative and attract more negativity when we can change our perception to focus on the positive, liberating ourselves and enabling us to reach a happier state of mind?

The subconscious mind LOVES to chat. Our thoughts are recited almost non-stop all day. The idea is to have realistic and productive inner monologues and not just brainwash ourselves with exaggerated positive remarks. Sometimes we really do need to "get real", realizing our mistakes and faults. We can use the setbacks we experience to learn from them and spring forward into action, to take us to where we were meant to be. The biggest mistake about making a mistake is not taking the lesson from it. See it as an opportunity to grow, and you will grow. Realistic thoughts are positive thoughts when they push you to achieve your goals. Continuous negative self-talk distracts, creates anxiety and prevents us from achieving our goals.

The route of all negativity is fear. Whether it is fear of loss, fear of getting hurt, worrying about the future — you name it — fear is the culprit. Did you know that 90 % of the things we worry about do not actually happen? Benjamin Franklin said, "Do not anticipate trouble or worry about what may never happen. Keep in the sunlight." So, why worry about things that are out of our control? Worrying incessantly and constantly ruminating in the negative is just wasted energy. We can't change anything by worrying. It would be far more fruitful and liberating to redirect this energy into using gratefulness as the antidote to being fearful. Identify the negative thought pattern immediately and switch focus to being grateful for the positives. What we see depends mainly on what we look for. If you tweak the way you look at things, what you look at can be altered or seen in an entirely new, positive light, with a brighter, more favourable outlook. There are ALWAYS positives if we search for them. Finding the positives in every situation, finding that silver lining and being grateful, makes you hopeful, thankful, optimistic and resilient. It also improves patience, sleep, and has been linked with less depression and anxiety.

Robert A. Emmons, PhD of the University of California and Michael E. McCullough of the University of Miami conducted research on the effects of gratitude on well-being. In the study, subjects journaled one sentence for five things they were grateful for, once a week. After only two months, there was a significant improvement in the subjects who made these written entries in their journal, compared to the control group. The group that expressed feelings of gratitude was happier, more optimistic and exercised more. Being grateful is instantly uplifting, and you can feel great!

It's easy to practice gratefulness if we overcome our biggest obstacle to being grateful, which is allowing ourselves to be sabotaged by negative thought patterns. MANY of our negative thoughts are actually irrational and affect our emotions. They are termed cognitive distortions.

Dr. Mike Dow, well-known psychotherapist and brain health expert, categorized them as 7 pitfall thought patterns: personalization, pervasiveness, pessimism, polarization, permanence, psychic and paralysis analysis. By being aware of these thought patterns, we can question them, change them and reshape our model of reality.

Here are some tips to stop giving energy to negative thoughts:

1) If something you perceive as negative happens, for example, after sending a long text to a friend anticipating a just-as-long reply, and you get a short, concise, seemingly blunt text. Don't go off on a tangent thinking, "Oh no, my text was probably so

silly. I am just not good at communicating and come across all wrong. I'm stupid. I should never speak my mind and type long texts." **Stop those thoughts (STT)**! Don't take things personally. Chances are your friend had a busy day, is tired or in a rush. Don't blame yourself. If we don't take things personally, we are more able to empathize with people and help bring about positive feelings of compassion — a better, more refreshing route. *Depersonalization* feels lighter. Choose to feel lighter.

2) If a small part of your day does not go according to plan, try not to let it filter through to alter the rest of your day. For example, after a late night and you're in a low mood, and then when you're up, you might be saying to yourself, "Oh no, this day is going to be terrible. I'm too tired. I might as well just sleep in all day." **Stop those thoughts (STT)**! Chances are, when you're up and moving and after having a brain-boosting breakfast, you can change the way you feel and have a day much better than you had expected. This is totally possible. Don't give in to hopelessness and helplessness. Choose to turn your day around. Do an activity without even thinking about it. We often give activities a lower rating when we are in a low mood and in a state of limiting beliefs before the activity, but after doing an activity, it's a given that we will feel much better.

Maybe do a quick run or some stretching exercises. Rate the activity after doing it, and be aware of the uplifting, energizing feelings the activity has given you. Remember THIS association the next time you're in a low mood and need to bounce back. Every moment is different. As the day progresses, things can change. Conquer *pervasiveness*.

3) Avoid catastrophic thinking. Believing the worst about everything and creating scenarios in your head about events

that may never occur will drain you. For example, "I didn't eat healthily today, so I'm going to become obese. I might as well never eat healthily again and give up." Again, question and challenge the validity of your thoughts. Is this really true? No. And how does it make you feel? Empowered? No. So, **stop those thoughts (STT)**! How about saying, "I didn't eat healthily today, but I will stay positive and strive to eat healthily from tomorrow onward. I will have more energy and a healthier mind and body." Now, doesn't that make you feel better? Your new feeling and new thinking will change your behaviour the next new day. Create your reality. *Stay positive.*

4) Living life in terms of absolutes — yes or no, seeing everything rigid, in black or white, is an example of all or nothing thinking. By being more accepting, tolerant and accommodating, we can avoid harsh emotions and stress-inducing mindsets. *Depolarize* yourself. Allow for flexibility in your thinking, and you will experience life as a rainbow of bright colour. Instead of thinking, "I didn't get a promotion this year; I might as well find another job." **Stop those thoughts** and rather think, "I didn't get a promotion this year, but I will work harder and maybe next year I will get a promotion."

Did you know that perfectionism is also a way of polarized thinking? Does everything have to be in exactly a certain order? Does everything really have to be perfect? Perfectionism in its maladaptive form can be unrealistic and can prevent you from being content in the moment while always striving to make things 100 % perfect. Perfection can be debilitating and can rob you of happiness.

5) I mentioned change in Chapter 1. Nothing is set in stone. Avoid making engraving remarks to yourself like, "I have always and will always eat tons of food when I am upset, sad or angry. I eat

for comfort and emotional eating is a part of myself and my future and, by the way, I'm sad and upset right now. Bring me some chocolate cake." *Nothing is permanent.* We can't change the past, but we can learn from it and impact our future by making the present bright.

Don't write yourself off. View challenging times as temporary, and it will pass. There IS a way out of dark, negative, thought patterns that alter your choices and behaviour. Just, you know, **stop those thoughts** (**STT**)! Life is going to present challenges, but you must persevere.

6) Don't make assumptions. *Don't assume* you know another person's thoughts and act on them. Acting on assumptions that aren't true can leave you feeling jolted and disappointed. "He didn't call. I think it's because I didn't sleep well when we met, and I looked like a bloated, tired zombie in my dress. Oh well — I think I should block his number now." Again, do we know for a fact that this is true? No. And how does this make you feel? Empowered? No! So, don't think about it that way. **Stop those thoughts! (STT)!** Mind reading and making assumptions can be unnecessarily harmful.

7) A series of negative irrational thoughts can often be never-ending and paralyzing if you get stuck in its negative loop. Surrender is the pathway to letting go. *Over-analysis* can steer you on a path to emotional paralysis. So, again, stop. Question your thoughts and break the negative cycle. We are our worst critics and can paralyze ourselves with self-defeating monologues. Don't be so hard on yourself. Have love and compassion for yourself. There's a quote by Jeff Brown that says "A better me is a better we." You have to make yourself happy first before you can make others happy. I know it may seem selfish, but it is quite the opposite. When you have love and compassion for yourself, you take care of yourself first and share the best

version of yourself with others, spreading the positive vibrations to others and enhance connections.

Bottom line, don't be a prisoner of your thoughts or other people's thoughts of you. Do not spend time worrying about what people think of you. Believe that you ARE ENOUGH, complete and whole on your own. Do not rely on affirmations from other people to validate who you are and you can be free and blissful.

Author and psychiatrist Dr. Daniel Amen mentions in his book, *Change your brain, change your life,* the 18:40:60 rule:

> When you are 18, you worry about what everyone thinks of you. When you are 40, you don't give a damn about what anybody thinks of you, and when you're 60, you realize that nobody has been thinking of you at all. People spend their days thinking about themselves, not you.

Another thought-provoking quote, to embed in our minds, by William James, "The greatest weapon against stress is our ability to choose one thought over another."

So, we now know how to identify negative thoughts and **stop those thoughts (STT)**. We also have the power to not only change our thinking but also transform our emotions and learn from them. Well-known author and psychiatrist, Dr. Judith Orloff, states that we can actually transform negative emotions with positive emotions. Fear can be transformed with courage. Jealousy and envy are transformed with self-esteem. Anger is transformed through empathy and compassion. Frustration can be transformed by practicing patience. Anxiety can be transformed with inner calm.

By being aware of negative thought patterns, we can identify their triggers and transform these negative emotions to positive ones. We know that we are mastering our emotions when we have patience and are less reactive. Take anger, for example. We can take a few slow and deep breaths, be patient until the thoughts pass through, practice empathy, love and compassion and respond rather than react with fiery charge. The sooner you let go of the anger, the more freedom from it you will have. This is a liberating truth. Another quote by Buddha, "Holding on to anger is like grasping hot coal with the intent of throwing it at someone else — you are the one that gets burned." Practice forgiveness not to condone another person's actions but to free yourself from negativity and positively wire your brain.

We can also adopt healthier mindsets and behaviours by changing the belief system of the subconscious "alter mind", by concentrating on the conscious mind. OK, so let's get conscious of these mindsets.

The conscious mind focuses mainly on information received from our five senses, and we use this part of our mind to think quickly and solve problems.

The subconscious mind contains information and belief systems created after years of conditioning. We are conditioned to believe or think in a certain way and, in doing so, act accordingly to what fits this model of reality. Whether it's via social media, advertisements or commercials, if we don't challenge what we see or hear, we begin to believe the ideas portrayed and form habits around them.

Constant exposure to something or repetition of a task can program the subconscious mind to do tasks automatically. Ever been on autopilot while driving the same route home daily — you're listening to the radio and not really thinking about the turns and suddenly you're home? That's your subconscious mind navigating you. The subconscious mind is the director of our habits. To change habits, we need to change the beliefs of our subconscious mind.

When we eat emotionally, for example, or have addictions to sugar, alcohol or any other substances, the conscious mind is well aware, "OK, just one chocolate bar, just one drink." The conscious mind is soon influenced by 4–7 thoughts transferred from the subconscious mind. So, basically, what's built in our subconscious mind dominates the conscious mind and will determine how we process new information.

This can alter decisions and lead to unhealthy choices, for example, "A few more chocolates will be comforting and make me feel happy," or "A few more drinks will make me fun and more sociable." Are these beliefs really true? Nope. After the havoc runs in the blood sugars from engorging on all that chocolate, you're bound to feel tired, lethargic and have a low mood. After all those drinks, it could eventually slow you down, reducing the fun and make socializing more difficult. Annie Grace, author of *This Naked Mind*, gives perfect examples in her book about dispelling conditioned beliefs.

For years and years we have been bombarded with unhealthy food and beverage commercials, and by constantly being exposed to it, we do not realize that we are transferring messages and thoughts from these commercials, into our brains, wiring the subconscious mind with beliefs and moulding our habits.

So, basically, habits form on a subconscious level and an empowering point to realize is that you can break unhealthy habits by rewiring your brain with positive messages. We do this by repetitively, positively affirming our conscious mind.

According to Dr. Caroline leaf, it takes 21 days for short-term memory to become long-term memory. It takes another 42 days, two more 21-day cycles, to turn it into a habit. It, therefore, takes 63 days to form a habit. The more you think about something, the more developed your memories surrounding the thought becomes.

Positive affirmations are powerful tools to transform your mind and work on both the conscious and subconscious mind. According to research, positive affirmations have the capacity to rewire our brains. When your brain has constant exposure to positive messages, your brain sees things in a positive way, and you become optimistic. Positive affirmations entrench new belief systems in your brain, along with better thoughts, to sprout better feelings and behaviours, which then will allow us to more likely achieve our goals and lead a healthier life.

Gary Hudson, author of *Positive Affirmations*, mentions in his book that positive affirmations keep the mind focused with better impulse control. There is a reduction in negative emotions, a better emotional regulation, an enhanced ability to focus and use strengths, and increase self-worth.

Research shows that positive thoughts promote self-esteem, and having high self-esteem helps people avoid problems with addictive behaviours such as emotional eating, smoking or drinking alcohol. Improving self-esteem is also vital in avoiding negative thoughts and negative energy in relationships.

OK, so by now, I am sure you're probably thinking, how do I stay positive and happy all the time and always expect everything great will always happen?

You don't have to be happy ALL the time, but when bad things happen, you will know that these dark patterns are temporary, that "this too shall pass," and you can have the skills to focus on the solution instead of on unhealthy mindsets, which can become programmed patterns in your brain. The key thing here is that you will be happier but, at the same time, realistic with a resilient mind. A resilient mind is better equipped to cope with stress; it's more adaptable, calm, caring, grounded, inspirational, peaceful and thoughtful.

Choose affirmations that will help you achieve a healthier life, mentally and physically and increase your well-being. Don't just visualize them, but write them down. Don't just say them, believe them. Don't just imagine them, feel them, and you will wire your brain to make things happen faster and feel great.

Say things like:

"I CAN DO IT, I CAN DO IT, I CAN DO IT."

"I will eat healthily for my mind."

"I will feed my brain with positive thoughts and nourishing food."

"I will reach my goal weight."

"I will control my blood sugars."

"I will conquer my mind."

"I will form healthy eating habits."

"I WILL be happy, healthy and mindful."

"Everything is possible."

"I am grateful for what I have."

"I am empowered to be the best version of myself."

A morning routine with positive affirmations will help bring down those barriers to change and wire your brain in a positive way. A quote from the book *The Secret*, "An affirmative thought is 100 times more powerful than a negative one." It will set the tone for the day, and you will more likely achieve your daily goals and, in time, you can change unhealthy habits. Barriers to change are imaginary. Upgrade your beliefs. Think in abundance.

Every day we are born again, and we should be grateful for it. Every day is a new beginning. Stay focused. You can rewire and train your brain. Have faith — it doesn't matter whether you believe in a superpower or not, but most importantly, have faith and belief in yourself. Hope is more powerful than fear. Don't lose hope. I love the proverb, "Just when the caterpillar thought its world was over, it became a butterfly."

CHAPTER 3

Nourish to Flourish.
Why Do We Need To Nourish The Brain?

Stop for a moment and be mindful of everything around you right now. Provoke your sense of wonder and take everything in as if you are seeing it all, for the very first time. The objects you see, the music you hear, the paintings on the wall, the smartphone in your pocket, the book on the table, the words that you're reading right now — everything around you was created from someone's imagination and is the result of that person's thoughts, streamed directly from their creative brain. This realization helps demonstrate how powerful the brain is and what it can achieve if we make the most of its magnifying potential.

Imagination and visualization are the magical ingredients to spark ideas, help one leap into action with passion and generate not just objects in the physical world but also amazing experiences. A healthy brain can help one relax to meditate peacefully, reflect, imagine and visualize dreams, bloom and burst with creativity and become insightful enough to improve intuition.

Every thought, every feeling and every movement we experience, from as small and as quick as the blink of an eye, are all controlled by the brain. In Chapter 2, we covered thoughts, feelings and positive affirmations. Staying positive, being grateful, having hope, faith, and belief, eliminating fear, experiencing love and joy are all made possible by our fascinating brain. The brain leads the mind and body and plays a role in everything we think and do. To optimize our minds, we need to optimize the health of our brain.

When our brains are healthy, we are more resilient and happier, and one of the best ways to keep our brain healthy is by feeding it healthy food. As the title of this chapter suggests, we need to nourish our brain to flourish.

Diet is a huge factor influencing brain health, partially because most of the brains structure is derived from food. Everything we eat and drink can have a profound impact on our brain, altering our thoughts, feelings, and behaviour, regardless of our age, gender or genetics. Take a moment and register that vital thought in your mind. All clear? Great. When we jump into proactive mode after experiencing a moment of clarity, we could spark a pivotal moment of change in our life. So, let's take action to nourish our brilliant brains the best we can, to actually BE the best we can. Our nutritional requirements need to be met so the conductor of our thoughts, feelings, and behaviour, can orchestrate most effectively.

So, how do we nourish our brain?

Want to know the brain's *recipe for vitality*? Here are the ingredients:

✓ Healthy omegas
✓ Complex carbohydrates
✓ Powerful proteins
✓ Energizing vitamins

      ✓   Magnificent minerals
      ✓   Waves of water (more on hydration in Chapter 7)

Each of these, above mentioned nutrition components, will have a distinct effect on brain functioning, development, mood, and energy. To understand how it all works, we need to first understand the brain, so let's explore the brain in this quick point-to-point tour.

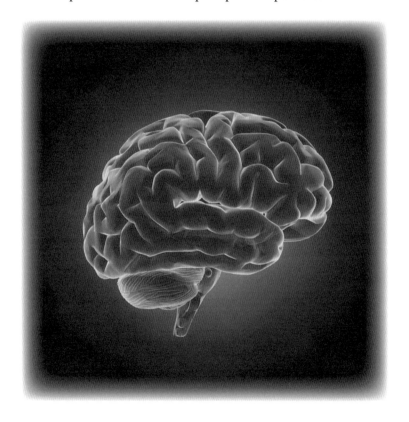

➢   The brain is home to over a 100 billion nerve cells. We call these nerve cells neurons.

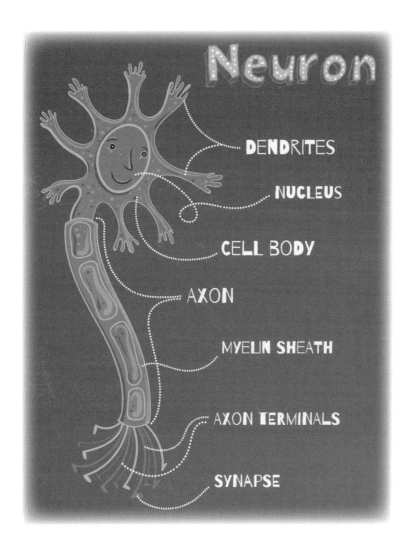

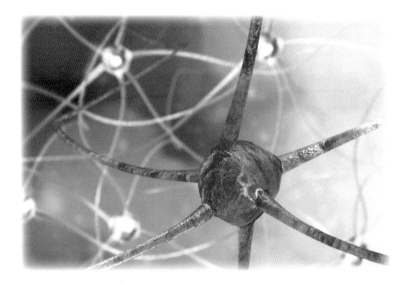

> Neurons connect with thousands of other neurons, forming an intricate neuronal network and communicate with each other through branches called dendrites.

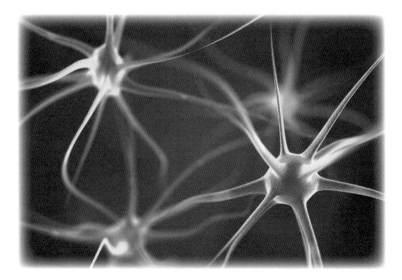

➤ Communication between these neurons takes place at junctions called synapses and is both electrical and chemical. Ever heard that famous question after meeting someone new, when people ask, "Was there any spark, any chemistry?" Well, there is, actually, some truth to this. The brain is all about electromagnetic fields, currents, impulses and waves producing chemical reactions, giving us these exciting feelings. Sparks really do fly.

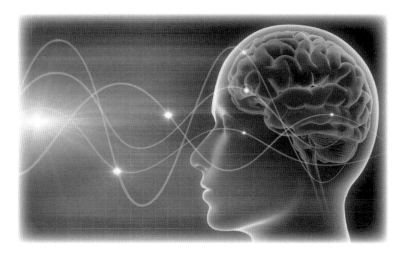

➤ When a neuron is stimulated, an electrical impulse is produced. Chemical messengers are then transmitted, at the synapse, from one neuron to the other.

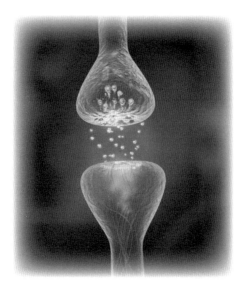

➢ We call these chemical messengers neurotransmitters, and there are many. For example, norepinephrine and epinephrine, gamma-amino-butyric acid (GABA), acetylcholine, dopamine and serotonin, all of these directly alter mood and functioning.

➢ The largest part of the brain is the cerebrum, which is divided into two hemispheres, connected by a bundle of nerve fibres called the corpus callosum.

➢ The cerebrum has four lobes: frontal, parietal, temporal, and occipital. Each lobe will produce a neurotransmitter affecting the way we feel. When we do not feel at our best, chances are our neurotransmitters are off-balance. When the brain is healthy, we usually produce balanced levels of neurotransmitters, and one of the ways to keep our brain healthy is by eating healthily.

Lobe to lobe, here are some quick brain basics in a nutshell.

Parts of the Human Brain

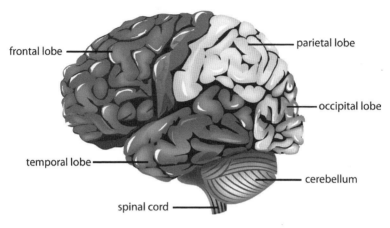

- Thinking about what to eat? Planning your meals? Finding reasons to attain your goals and trying to understand, make sense of, and conquer obstacles to achieve them? Thinking, planning, reasoning, understanding: this is the **frontal lobe** of your brain guiding you in action. The frontal lobe also plays a role in emotions and controls voluntary muscles in your body, helping you move.

✓ The neurotransmitter dopamine is produced in the frontal lobe and gives us a sense of pleasure and reward. It also influences sleep, learning, and behaviour. When we do not produce enough dopamine, we lose our drive and motivation, and our thinking, planning, and reasoning depreciate.

- Sensory information from reading a recipe, recognizing languages ("bon appetite"), to tasting

33

and touching delectable food and keeping oriented in this way, is **the parietal lobe** of the brain in action.

✓ Acetylcholine is the neurotransmitter produced in this lobe and is a building block of the myelin sheath, a protective insulating layer around neurons. We also need this neurotransmitter to improve memory, keep us alert, attentive and razor sharp. Acetylcholine also plays a role in learning, modulates communication and helps us respond to sensory stimuli.

• You hear the succulent steak sizzle on the barbeque stand. The sounds of sautéing chicken on the stove. You ask yourself, "Is my delicious dinner ready to be devoured as yet?" **The temporal lobe** of the brain is responsible for all this auditory information as well as visual recognition. The temporal lobe is also used for learning, memory and helps us makes sense of and respond to questions, "Why do I need to eat healthily? Oh, I know – I want to have tons of energy, eat well, feel well, exercise well and sleep well."

✓ The neurotransmitter called Gamma aminobutyric acid (GABA) is produced in this lobe. GABA is known for its calming and relaxing sensations.

• **The occipital lobe** is responsible for visual perception. Everything your eyes take in, from the shapes and colours of food to the environment around you, the ambience and people present in a restaurant, for example. These are the activities of the occipital lobe.

✓ Serotonin is the neurotransmitter produced in this lobe and is known for its effects on mood, sleep, and memory. Serotonin also alters appetite and an imbalance can lead to sugar cravings. When you're craving those delicious desserts stop for a moment and ask yourself, "What emotion am I feeling? Am I sad and down?" Often serotonin levels may be low and when we have correct levels of serotonin we feel great. Bottom line, serotonin is the happy neurotransmitter, often known to banish the blues.

➢ The neurotransmitters, norepinephrine along with epinephrine (adrenalin) are responsible for the fight-or-flight response. When we are stressed out or feel threatened in a situation, these neurotransmitters increase our heart rate and blood sugars and increases blood flow to muscles, preparing us to leap into action in an attempt to help us cope.

So, what was the point of all this neurotransmitter jargon? Let's transmit this idea to both our short-term and long-term memory — A healthy brain produces healthy levels of neurotransmitters. We need to eat healthily to have a healthy brain.

Flourish with Protein:
Why Does the Brain Need Protein?

Proteins are broken down to amino acids, which are the building blocks of the neurotransmitters mentioned earlier, which strongly impact the way we feel and behave. Essential amino acids are termed *essential* as the body cannot make these amino acids on its own. It would need to be derived from our diet to alter the way we feel.

If we do not consume sufficient amounts of amino acids from our diet, we will be unable to produce the blue banishing serotonin or the get our motivation and drive from pleasurable dopamine. For example, the amino acid tryptophan (which we get from turkey, eggs, lean meat, and beans) is converted to 5-hydroxytryptophan (5-HTP), which is required to produce serotonin and serotonin is used to produce the sleep-enhancing melatonin, vital for rest and well-being. We cannot produce dopamine, noradrenaline, and adrenalin without adequate amounts of the amino acid tyrosine, and we cannot produce acetylcholine without choline.

Flourish with Fats:
Why are Fats Essential for the Brain?

There's the term again, "essential fats". Essential fats are fats that cannot be produced by the body and must be derived from the diet. Our brains need these healthy fats and as a matter of "fat" did you know that 60 % of our brains is actually composed of fats.

Omega-3 essential fatty acids and omega-6 essential fatty acids comprise 20 % of the fats in our brain and are crucial to maintain the fluidity and flexibility of neuron membranes. We want our neuron membranes to be fluid so that neurons can communicate easily with each other. Omega-3 fatty acids, in particular (from oily fish, nuts, and seeds), prevent the myelin sheath (the insulating layer around neurons), from becoming rigid and allows for smooth communication between neurons.

As with anything in life, what you put in is what you will get out. If we want our brain to work optimally we need to fuel it with healthy fats. Consumption of unhealthy fats from deep-fried foods and commercially prepared baked goods compete with essential fats in the brain and increase the rigidity of neuron membranes. So, basically just imagine that unhealthy fats make neuron membranes solid, almost like building a brick wall around neurons making communication with each other difficult.

Another fat or *lipid* called phospholipids (found in eggs and organ meat) is required to make neurotransmitter receptor sites and the protective myelin sheath. As we age, the myelin sheath around neurons can wear down slowing communication between neurons. We need to maintain brain cell membranes keeping them flexible with healthy fats so our brains can function well.

Flourish with Complex Carbohydrate: Why does the Brain Need Complex Carbs?

There's tons of hype out there about carbohydrates being super bad and should be eliminated completely. We don't have to banish all carbs, just the refined highly processed carbs such as white breads, processed cereals, and products made with white flour. These are carbs that are digested faster and cause a rapid release of sugar in the blood and glucose to brain. The brain does require glucose for fuel but not elevated levels. We don't want rapid spikes in blood sugars but a more gradual slow release of glucose to the brain.

Complex carbs such as whole grains, beans, and vegetables are digested slower and cause a gradual release of glucose to the brain. Complex carbs will be made simple when we get clued up on the carbs to choose and the carbs to curb, in the next chapter.

Flourish with Vitamins and Minerals: Why Does the Brain Need Vitamins and Minerals?

We mentioned the role of fats, proteins and complex carbs for the brain. Well, without vitamins and minerals these nutrition components cannot perform their roles effectively. Vitamins and minerals work as cofactors and take part in many enzymatic reactions in the body. Cofactors are helper molecules that your body needs to help convert carbohydrates to glucose for fuel, help amino acids form neurotransmitters and manoeuvre the fats we eat to cell membranes in the brain. Some vitamins and minerals are also antioxidants and protect the brain from oxidative damage. A deficiency in vitamins and minerals is sometimes implicated in a number of mental health problems. More on vitamin and mineral deficiencies will be coming up in the next chapter.

Take-away point to "absorb" from this chapter: Nourishing the brain with the right type of carbohydrates, essential fats, amino acids, vitamins, and minerals is essential for heightened functioning of the brain and will enable you to flourish.

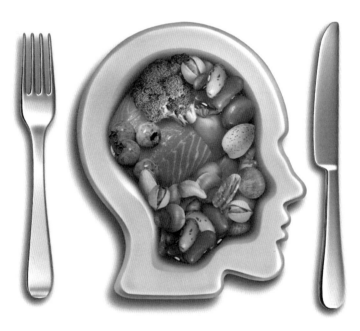

CHAPTER 4

Recharge, Reboot, Rejuvenate, Elevate – Conquer the Culprits

Do you often feel tired and lethargic? Have a depressed mood? Feeling anxious? Addicted? Have trouble with ADHD? We have already established, thus far, that what you eat will alter the way you feel. The emerging field of nutritional psychiatry is relatively new and explores the association between diet quality and mental health.

In Chapter 3, we discussed how amino acids from our diet are used to make the neurotransmitters serotonin, dopamine, adrenaline, noradrenalin, acetylcholine and GABA. An imbalance or lack of any of these neurotransmitters may leave us feeling anxious, tired and lethargic with a low mood, a lack of motivation and drive.

Let's be mindful of the brain on food and go through the culprits that alter neurotransmitter balance or hamper your mood, concentration, focus, sleep, energy, and well-being.

4.1 Culprit alert! Sugar

The Brain on Sugar and Other Addictive Substances – The "Not So Sweet" Cycle

The amount of sugar you eat can directly impact your mood, level of relaxation, alertness, memory, and sleep. The more unstable your blood sugars, the more you will experience symptoms of fatigue, dizziness, irritability, poor concentration and depression.

When we devour a sweet dessert or any other addictive substance such as alcohol, a signal is sent to the cerebral cortex of the brain, and the brain's reward system is activated. The brain's reward system is a series of chemical and electrical pathways that lead our subconscious mind to make an association between what we are consuming and the satisfying feeling produced after consuming it.

A high consumption of sugar increases the neurotransmitter called dopamine. When dopamine is released, you feel uplifted and rewarded initially, but about 1-2 hours later you may notice yourself feeling down, foggy, drowsy and irritable. If you keep pushing the brain to release dopamine with more sugar, alcohol or any other addictive substance, the brain responds by down-regulating dopamine receptors to stop producing natural dopamine. These low levels of dopamine lead to symptoms of lethargy, lack of motivation, and drive.

Frequent high consumption of sugar results in tolerance and withdrawal, which are the hallmarks of addiction. Addiction is a strong word but helps us realize the power certain foods can have on our brain. You may crave more sugar to give you the same heightened feeling after developing a tolerance and will feel withdrawal symptoms such as fatigue, lethargy, low mood and headaches if sugar is not consumed in these amounts.

I often see many patients with low energy levels, poor sleep, heightened levels of anxiety, mood imbalances with intense cravings, and after a detailed dietary history, I often find sugar a contributing factor to the roller coaster of emotions. Mindlessly craving sugar and satisfying these cravings by engorging chocolate, desserts, processed carbohydrates, one may not realize the developing addiction to sugar. Did you know that sugar is said to be about eight times more addictive than cocaine? Falling into the sugar addiction cycle can lead to a host of health problems such as obesity, diabetes, cardiovascular disease, depression, and poor sleep.

As with many addictions, initially, cravings are satisfying, blood pressure, heart rate, and energy levels increase. Insulin increases to stabilize blood sugars and when blood sugars drop shortly afterwards, there is often irritability, anxiety, lack of patience and eventually fatigue and lethargy. The stress hormone cortisol is then increased, which can make one feel even more anxious, panicky and unsettled, initiating further cravings as seen in withdrawal. We can prevent these feelings by controlling our blood sugars and wisely choosing LOW glycemic index complex carbs (explained soon).

We mentioned in the previous chapter, the brain does need glucose for fuel — not elevated sugar spikes but a more gradual release of glucose to the brain. Avoiding refined, highly processed carbohydrates and choosing to eat healthier complex carbohydrates achieves this. So, let's equip ourselves with ways to control blood sugars and avoid those unpleasant blood sugar surges as imbalances are definitely no joke.

There is a great tool used in dietary practice called the **glycemic index,** which measures how much a food boosts blood sugars after consuming it. Simply put, high glycemic index carbohydrates result in a rapid release of sugar into the blood and a quick spike in insulin (a hormone secreted by the pancreas to help control blood sugars). High GI foods tend to cause a crash after the spike in blood sugars, altering mood, and increase appetite and cravings.

Figure 1: Blood Sugar Response Curves For High GI And Low GI Foods

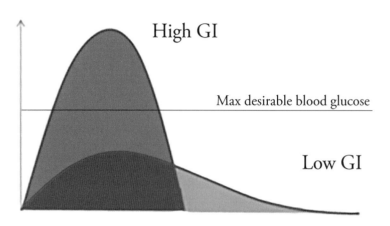

Low glycemic index foods, on the other hand, cause a more gradual release of sugar in the blood, improve satiety and produce a more sustainable supply of energy over a longer time. Bottom line, we want to prevent the peaks and valleys in blood sugars for better mood, energy and to prevent cravings.

Generally, foods with fibre have a lower GI and are great choices. Fibre in a food delays the digestion of sugar, causing it to be released slowly. When buying foods, take a look at the ingredients list and look for the items that have at least 4 g of fibre per serving. Fibre will also make you feel full faster and equip you with energy over a longer period of time, so let's get into a fibre frenzy and fibre away!

Not sure whether a food is LOW GI or HIGH GI? Just look at it. Does it look white and plain — made from white flour, white breads? Is it highly processed and refined? Would it break up easily in water or milk? The faster a food can break down, the faster it would be digested and, in doing so, will cause a rapid release of sugar into the blood. Cornflakes in milk, for example. Cornflakes become mushy quickly and break up easily and are, therefore, a HIGH GI carb. An easy way to remember: HH (High GI = higher blood sugars). If a food is brown, seedy and granular, requiring lots of chewing and has fibre such as beans, lentils, steel-cut oats, they are more likely to be LOW GI: LL (Low GI = lower blood sugars).

So, let's apply the GI and shift our minds to switch:

➢ HIGH GI white bread with LOWER GI multigrain bread
➢ HIGH GI cornflakes and processed cereals with LOWER GI steel-cut oats
➢ HIGH GI baked potato or mashed potato with LOWER GI sweet potato
➢ HIGH GI French fries with LOWER GI yam fries (baked)
➢ HIGH GI corn with LOWER GI peas
➢ HIGH GI white rice with LOWER GI brown and wild rice, beans, and lentils

GI idea "Engrained" in your head? Great.

Most fruit and vegetables are LOW GI especially green leafy vegetables and fruit with a skin or peel. An apple, for example, even though it contains sugar, has fibre in the peel of the apple and this delays the digestion of the sugar. Fruit without a skin or peel such as melons and litchi will cause a rapid sugar spike as it lacks fibre, causing us to crave more sweet foods shortly after consuming them.

Remember, having variety, moderation and balance is key, so even though LOW GI carbs are the way to go, we always want to watch our portions. Too much of anything at once can affect the way we feel and cause us to gain weight, and the weight gain can eventually lead to an increase in blood sugars causing more insulin to be secreted. Guess what? Did you know that insulin is also a fat storing hormone and often contributes to further weight gain?

With all the weight gain, one can eventually become insulin resistant where insulin no longer works and blood sugars remain elevated. That's NOT sweet at all, so let's "insulate" ourselves against the sweetness. Also, don't forget what we learned from Chapter 1, the more overweight a person is, the smaller the memory centre of their brain.

When excess glucose binds to protein in the brain through a process called glycation, beta-amyloid protein plaques form in the brain, altering memory, as seen in Alzheimer's disease. By the way, researchers are now beginning to call Alzheimer's disease Type 3 diabetes for this reason, so guard your memory by keeping your blood sugars in check.

According to well-known nutrition expert Patrick Holford, glucose itself is not toxic, provided you can keep your blood sugars even. An excess of glucose becomes toxic to the brain, causing inflammation and damage to nerve cells, preventing them from working properly. Brain neuron membranes become thicker and communication between neurons is slowed. Studies have found that high sugar consumption has been implicated in aggressive behaviour, anxiety, hyperactivity, depression, eating disorders and fatigue.

So, no "sugar coating",. Sugar is definitely a culprit and needs to be avoided. Be wary of food labels and ingredient lists at the back of a product as this culprit is out to control us. Try not to choose products that have more than seven ingredients in the ingredient list. The more ingredients a product has, chances are it's more refined and highly processed. The shorter the ingredients list, the better.

Be mindful that words appearing in an ingredient list appear in order of quantity or amount, with the highest amount used in the product, at the beginning of the list.

If you see sugar listed in the first five words of the ingredients list, know that this product has lots of sugar and will have an effect on your blood sugars.

I often see patients with elevated blood sugar levels, who state that they do not consume any white sugar or brown sugar, but after completing a dietary history I find that they are taking in hidden sources of sugar.

Some words in the ingredients list to avoid are pretty straightforward:

+ white sugar
+ brown sugar
+ invert sugar
+ cane sugar

Be wary of all words in an ingredients list ending in "ose" as these will increase blood sugars:

+ glucose
+ lactose
+ maltose
+ sucrose
+ fructose

Other words to look out for include:

+ syrups such as corn syrup, maple syrup, brown rice syrup, agave syrup
+ maltodextrin
+ honey
+ molasses
+ barley malt
+ crystals
+ concentrate

You're probably wondering, "Why is fructose on the list? Fructose is from fruit. Why is fructose on the list, but we can still have apples and blueberries?" And then the famous question, "Can I add fruit juices to my smoothies?"

Here's the answer: We mentioned earlier that fibre delays the digestion of sugar, causing a slower release of sugar in the blood. Fruit with a skin or peel will have fibre, which delays the digestion of fructose in the fruit (mentioned earlier). Fruit juices are highly concentrated, loaded with sugar and don't have enough fibre to delay the sugar release, resulting in rapid peaks and valleys in blood sugars shortly after consuming it. Ever notice with fruit juice, there is often a vicious cycle of thirst for more fruit juice shortly afterwards? This is because of the sugar spike and subsequent crash it creates, sending you on a sweet treasure hunt for more sweet items.

Check the nutrient label: A 100 g serving size of a product should not have more than 5 g of sugar. If an item says "No Sugar Added", it actually means there is enough sugar in the product as it is and more sugar did not have to be added. It is NOT a sugar-free or *guilt-free* product. Opt for sugar-free, unsweetened varieties.

This brings me to my next point about artificial sweeteners and the question, "Are artificial sweeteners good substitutes for sugar?" It was yes. This is no longer true. According to functional medicine specialist Dr. Vincent Pedre, artificial sweeteners are now known to overstimulate your sweet receptors, so you cannot appreciate the sweetness in berries, for example. One would crave sweeter foods and cause blood sugar and insulin spikes. Artificial sweeteners are now known to disturb the bacteria in our gut, which can alter mood (more bacteria talk in the next chapter). Aspartame, an artificial sweetener, is a neurotoxin (a toxin that can cause damage to nerve tissue). If you want to use a sweetener, try a natural sweetener like Stevia or use cinnamon in your tea or coffee. Another option is to surrender the sweetness completely and choose turmeric, ginger or lemon in your tea.

When having a meal that could raise your blood sugar, a good trick would be to add vinegar to your salads and have your vegetables before consuming the foods that could cause a blood sugar spike.

A study published in the *European Journal of Clinical Nutrition* showed that vinegar supplementation lowers glucose, and insulin responses and can increase satiety in a meal. Vinegar helped lower the GI of a bread meal in healthy volunteers. Apple cider vinegar, white vinegar, and balsamic vinegar are great choices.

4.2 Culprit alert! Gluten

Foggy About Gluten? Gluten-free Made Easy

We have all come across the term *gluten-free* while grocery shopping or eating out — the term is widespread. So, what is gluten, and what is all the hype about being gluten-free?

Gluten is an insoluble protein composite consisting of two proteins (glutenin and gliadin) and is found in certain grains, particularly wheat, barley, and rye.

It has been well documented for years that a gluten-free diet has been recommended for people with wheat allergy and Celiac disease (an inherited disease in which gluten consumption may cause inflammation of the lining of the small intestine, leading to gastrointestinal discomfort, nutrient malabsorption and bone loss).

New research is showing that a large population of people can now become sensitive to gluten without having Celiac disease. People with *non-Celiac gluten sensitivity* may also experience bloating, digestive disturbances, fatigue, headaches, and joint pain after gluten is consumed.

We are all aware of the gastrointestinal side effects after eating gluten such as: bloating, diarrhea or constipation and stomach pain. Recent research has now focused on the effects of gluten consumption on the brain. Dr. David Perlmutter, well-known neurologist, mentions in his book *Grain brain,* an editorial from the *Journal of Neurology, Neurosurgery and Psychiatry* called "Gluten sensitivity as a neurological illness" by Dr. Hadjivassiliou and his team, who concluded that people can have issues with brain function without having any gastrointestinal problems whatsoever.

According to Dr. Vincent Pedre, author of *Happy Gut,* partially digested gluten forms proteins (called gliadorphins, also known as gluteomorphins), which react with opium receptors in the brain, mimicking the effects of opiate drugs like morphine and heroin. These compounds affect the temporal lobe area of the brain associated with speech and hearing comprehension.

What you eat and the ecosystem of your gut determines how your gut will function (more about this in the next chapter). Bi-directional communication occurs via the gut and the brain (the gut-brain axis), and signals from the gut to the brain can be inflammatory in nature. Improperly digested gluten can trigger the immune system, causing inflammation in the gut. Inflammation in the gut is linked to inflammation in the brain, causing one to feel fatigued, cloudy and feel symptoms of anxiety and depression as well as other behavioural and mental problems. After eating a heavy, gluten-containing meal, one would feel tired and lethargic, have headaches, reduced mental clarity and an inability to focus.

The word gluten is actually derived from Latin meaning glue, describing its sticky and difficult to digest nature. The following is a list from the Canadian Celiac Association, which indicate the presence of gluten in a food item.

Stick these words in your head and be mindful of them when browsing the ingredients list.

- Barley (flakes, flour, pearl)
- Atta (chapatti flour)
- Beer, ale, lager
- Bread and bread stuffing
- Brewer's yeast
- Bulgur
- Couscous
- Croutons
- Dinkel (also known as spelt)
- Durum
- Einkorn
- Emmer
- Farina
- Farro
- Fu
- Graham flour
- Hydrolyzed wheat protein
- Kamut
- Malt, malt extract, malt syrup, and malt flavouring
- Malt vinegar
- Malt milk
- Modified wheat starch
- Oatmeal, oat bran, oat flour, rolled oats (unless from pure uncontaminated oats)
- Pasta
- Rye bread and flour
- Seitan (a meat-like food derived from wheat gluten, used in many vegetarian dishes, sometimes called "wheat meat")
- Triticale
- Wheat bran
- Wheat flour
- Wheat germ
- Wheat starch

Yes, this list is long as this culprit lurks in many foods, but it's not as daunting and restrictive as you think. I often hear patients say, "So, what can I eat?" There are many gluten-free options available.

Gluten-free made easy — Here's a list of gluten-free options:

✓ All fruit
✓ All vegetables
✓ Meat, fish, poultry, eggs, dairy
✓ Beans, peas, lentils, chickpeas
✓ Nuts and seeds
✓ Grains such as amaranth, arrowroot, buckwheat, corn, bran, millet, quinoa, rice (brown and wild, basmati, red, jasmine, white rice), rice crackers, sorghum flour, sweet potato flour, tapioca
✓ Oats (pure only — beware of cross-contamination, though, if made in an industry surrounded by other gluten-containing grains)
✓ Fats and oils (avocado, olive, canola)
✓ Tea, coffee, distilled alcohol (bourbon, rum, gin, rye, whisky, scotch, vodka, pure liqueurs)
✓ Condiments and spices (pickles, relish, olives, ketchup, mustard, tomato paste, pure herbs and spices, black pepper, salt, vinegars such as apple cider, rice, balsamic, distilled white, grape, rice or wine)

On another "sticky" note, let's remember to opt for the LOW GI, high fibre varieties (discussed earlier). Avoid the refined gluten-free options as it could spike blood sugar and affect the way we feel.

So, what is the verdict? Gluten impacts our mind far more than previously thought. When it comes to healthy eating, variety, moderation, and balance are key components, but if you're mindful of what you eat — your brain will thank you.

4.3 Culprit alert! Deficiencies

Feeling Low?
Maybe You're Not Getting Enough of the Good Stuff?

If we want to feel uplifted and resilient, we need to make sure we are getting optimal amounts of the right nutrients daily. Vitamins and minerals alter the way we feel and are used to produce a steady supply of neurotransmitters. A lack of vital nutrients and too few neurotransmitters can produce negative and counterproductive mind-altering states.

When it comes to vitamin and mineral supplements, "food first" is a dietitian motto for sure. A well-balanced diet, which includes a rainbow of colourful fruit and vegetables can provide vital vitamins and minerals required for good health and well-being. Unfortunately, many of us don't eat as well as we should with our busy schedules and hectic lifestyles, often skipping meals, and research indicates that a supplement could be necessary to ensure our nutritional requirements are met.

People who eliminate whole food groups or follow restrictive diets to lose weight or manage allergies, as well as those doing intermittent fasting, require supplementation to prevent low levels of vitamins and minerals.

It is best to speak to a registered dietitian for advice on your nutritional requirements as everyone is unique and has different nutritional needs depending on their age, gender, medical condition, medication, and lifestyle. Let's explore why we need enough of the good stuff and the foods you can get them from.

Not Enough Vitamin B 12?

We have all had those sudden quick lapses in short-term memory. Ever forget where you placed your keys? Went into a room to get an item but the item you were looking for suddenly slipped your mind? What about forgetting where you parked your car? Do these sudden brain fog experiences sound familiar? The frequency of these forgetful symptoms could be your brain's way of "reminding" you that you may not be getting enough vitamin B12 (also known as Cobalamin).

Vitamin B12 plays an essential role in the normal functioning of the brain and the nervous system. It is required to manufacture neurotransmitters (the chemical messengers in the brain) and produce the myelin sheath (the insulating layer found around nerves), which allows electrical impulses to transmit messages quickly and efficiently along nerve cells.

A lack of vitamin B12 in your diet or poor absorption of the vitamin could cause mental fog, affect your memory and dampen your mood. Depression is actually a common symptom of vitamin B12 deficiency. The role of vitamin B12 in mental health is expanding, and this valuable vitamin is now known to be vital in maintaining brain mass and preventing brain shrinkage often associated with dementia.

Ever had a good long sleep but not rejuvenated or revitalized when you're up? Instead of waking up well rested, you find yourself feeling tired, wanting to sleep more? Sound familiar? Confusing right? It is important to note that consuming insufficient amounts of vitamin B12 can often lead to a marked decrease in energy levels, even if not sleep deprived. Vitamin B12 helps blood carry oxygen in the body (which is essential for energy), and it is also required to form red blood cells. A deficiency of vitamin B12 can cause anemia, making you feel tired and lethargic. Other symptoms of vitamin B12 deficiency include weakness, light-headedness, a numbness or a tingling-like sensation in extremities, muscle fatigue, and hair loss.

The absorption of vitamin B12 requires *intrinsic factor* (produced with stomach acid). As we get older, our stomach produces less acid and insufficient amounts of intrinsic factor, making us more prone to deficiency. Medication that decrease the secretion of stomach acid such as antacids, antihistamines, proton-pump inhibitors, and even some diabetes medication such as Metformin, can decrease the absorption of vitamin B12 and increase the risk of deficiency.

Alcohol and other substances are also known to deplete B vitamins including vitamin B12, contributing to deficiencies, affecting mood and altering the memory centres in the brain, making supplementation with B vitamins essential. Vegetarians, vegans or anyone at risk of vitamin B12 deficiency require supplementation with sublingual vitamin B12 or vitamin B12 shots.

Vitamin B12, together with other B vitamins such as folic acid, can help keep your homocysteine levels in check. An elevated homocysteine level is associated with an increased risk for cardiovascular diseases and depression.

Where do we find it?

- ✓ Meat
- ✓ Poultry
- ✓ Fish
- ✓ Eggs
- ✓ Oysters
- ✓ Lamb
- ✓ Liver
- ✓ Fortified cereals
- ✓ Shitake mushrooms

Not Enough Vitamin B1 (Thiamin)?

A lack of vitamin B1 can alter memory, concentration, cause anxiety and irritability, mental and physical tiredness. We need this key nutrient to convert food to energy and keep us feeling energetic. Research shows that supplementing with vitamin B1 can leave one feeling clearheaded and composed, with faster reaction times. An important point to remember is that this vitamin, crucial for brain health, is easily depleted with alcohol consumption, which can often lead to a condition called Wernicke-Korsakoff syndrome, giving one symptoms of depression, anxiety, confusion and loss of memory.

When drinking alcohol, definitely supplement with Thiamin. So, vitamin B1 — is it the one and only? Nope, not so. When taking a single B vitamin, it's best to take it with a multivitamin or B complex vitamin as B vitamins work best when taken together.

Where do we find it?

- ✓ Watercress
- ✓ Asparagus
- ✓ Brussel sprouts
- ✓ Peas
- ✓ Lettuce
- ✓ Peppers
- ✓ Cabbage
- ✓ Cauliflower
- ✓ Mushrooms
- ✓ Beans
- ✓ Whole grains
- ✓ Squash
- ✓ Soy milk
- ✓ Tomatoes
- ✓ Lentils
- ✓ Nuts and seeds

✓ Oats
✓ Liver
✓ Mussels

Not Enough Vitamin B2 (Riboflavin)?

Vitamin B2, as with all B vitamins, is also important as a cofactor to convert fats, sugars, and protein to energy and, in doing so, boost your energy levels. It may also help protect cells from oxidative damage. Make sure you get enough B2 for a better you.

Where do we find it?

✓ Milk
✓ Yogurt
✓ Cheese
✓ Whole grains
✓ Liver
✓ Mushrooms
✓ Watercress
✓ Cabbage
✓ Asparagus
✓ Broccoli
✓ Pumpkin
✓ Bean sprouts
✓ Mackerel
✓ Tomatoes
✓ Spinach
✓ Lamb
✓ Almonds
✓ Salmon
✓ Eggs

Not Enough Vitamin B3 (Niacin)?

The brain and nervous system need vitamin B3 to thrive. It's also essential for healthy skin and blood cells. Without B3, one would experience deficiency symptoms of anxiety, depression, irritability, poor memory, difficulty sleeping, headaches and as with all B vitamin deficiencies — lack of energy.

Niacin is also known to help balance blood sugars and cholesterol levels. Vitamin B3 can be made from the amino acid tryptophan, but guess what? We need those complex carbs I mentioned earlier to make tryptophan more available to us to be used properly. So, if you're doing turkey, it wouldn't hurt to do some whole grains with it to maximize the tryptophan to serotonin to melatonin conversion or, in other words, to feel good and sleep well.

Where do we find it?

- ✓ Salmon
- ✓ Chicken
- ✓ Tuna
- ✓ Mushrooms
- ✓ Whole grains
- ✓ Peanut butter
- ✓ Cabbage
- ✓ Asparagus
- ✓ Lamb
- ✓ Tomatoes
- ✓ Squash
- ✓ Cauliflower
- ✓ Peanuts
- ✓ Turkey
- ✓ Liver
- ✓ Avocado
- ✓ Peas
- ✓ Grass-fed beef

Not Enough Vitamin B5 (Pantothenic acid)?

Feeling stressed and need a helping hand? Let's "high five" vitamin B5! Pantothenic acid helps makes anti-stress hormones, so without it, we feel…? Yes, you guessed it — stressed, along with having poor memory and concentration as it plays a role in producing the neurotransmitter acetylcholine required for these functions.

The brain and nerves need B5, and a deficiency would give us symptoms of anxiety, tiredness, and exhaustion, especially after exercise. The good news about this vitamin is that it is easily available in a variety of foods. Very easy to get.

Where do we find it?

- ✓ Chicken
- ✓ Whole grains
- ✓ Broccoli
- ✓ Avocados
- ✓ Mushrooms
- ✓ Tomatoes
- ✓ Watercress
- ✓ Peas
- ✓ Lentils
- ✓ Cabbage
- ✓ Celery
- ✓ Strawberries
- ✓ Eggs
- ✓ Squash
- ✓ Salmon
- ✓ Shellfish
- ✓ Meat

Not Enough Vitamin B6 (Pyridoxine)?

Remember the blue banishing serotonin we mentioned in earlier chapters? Well, without B6, we can't convert amino acid tryptophan to serotonin, which also means, as we know by now, our mood and sleep would be affected. Other known deficiencies of serotonin manifest in depression, irritability, stress, nervousness and lack of energy from all that lack of sleep. So, basically, we cannot produce sleep-inducing melatonin without serotonin. On top of that, B6 helps reduce homocysteine levels along with B12 and folic acid. We also need B6 to make red blood cells and gain energy to do the things we love to do, like take that quick run to build neurons. Being a diuretic, B6 also helps reduce bloating and is known to be helpful in alleviating premenstrual syndrome symptoms (PMS). Oral contraceptives deplete B6, which is a cofactor for feel-good serotonin and GABA, so make sure you supplement if taking these meds.

Let's throw some B6 into our nutrient mix.

Where do we find it?

- ✓ Asparagus
- ✓ Lentils
- ✓ Bananas
- ✓ Cauliflower
- ✓ Meat
- ✓ Poultry
- ✓ Chickpeas
- ✓ Beans
- ✓ Onions
- ✓ Broccoli
- ✓ Peppers
- ✓ Cabbage
- ✓ Brussel sprouts
- ✓ Tofu

- ✓ Salmon
- ✓ Tuna
- ✓ Cottage cheese
- ✓ Nuts
- ✓ Squash

Not Enough Vitamin C?

Let's "C" what this vitamin does for mental health. Vitamin C, this powerful antioxidant (and more about antioxidants later) is also needed to make the neurotransmitter serotonin, and studies have linked a deficiency to depression. Much more about collagen later, but what I love to mention is that vitamin C works with this anti-aging protein to keep not only our hair, skin, and nails healthy but also improve gut symptoms and help us sleep. The body does not make vitamin C on its own or store it, so best to ensure you're getting enough vitamin C from your diet to experience the benefits.

Where do we find it?

- ✓ Broccoli
- ✓ Brussel sprouts
- ✓ Citrus fruit
- ✓ Bell peppers
- ✓ Spinach
- ✓ Strawberries
- ✓ Tomatoes
- ✓ Cauliflower
- ✓ Cabbage
- ✓ Sweet potato
- ✓ Squash

Not Enough Folic Acid, Vitamin B9?

Folic acid deficiency can leave you anxious and depressed, have poor memory and alter your appetite, giving you lack of concentration and energy. This vitamin is world famous for preventing brain and spinal birth defects when taken early in pregnancy and is needed to create new cells.

Along with B12 and B6, as mentioned earlier, folic acid can lower homocysteine levels. Another deficiency symptom is anemia, as folic acid is needed to make red blood cells. Bottom line — if you want to feel revitalized and energetic, follow up with folic acid and dine with B9.

Where do we find it?

- ✓ Asparagus
- ✓ Spinach
- ✓ Turnip
- ✓ Broccoli
- ✓ Kale
- ✓ Brussel sprouts
- ✓ Romaine lettuce
- ✓ Citrus fruit
- ✓ Celery
- ✓ Lentils
- ✓ Black eyes peas
- ✓ Beans
- ✓ Chickpeas
- ✓ Tomato juice
- ✓ Walnuts
- ✓ Avocados
- ✓ Cauliflower
- ✓ Okra
- ✓ Beets

Not Enough Vitamin D?

This sunshine vitamin could definitely help "brighten" up your days and keep the dark shadows of low mood at bay. Deficiencies of vitamin D have been linked to seasonal affective disorder, anxiety, depression, and dementia.

Where do we find it?

✓ Salmon
✓ Tuna
✓ Sardines
✓ Mackerel
✓ Herring
✓ Trout
✓ Eggs
✓ Mushrooms
✓ Cottage cheese

Not Enough Vitamin E?

We need vitamin E to help reverse oxidative damage to cells and neuron membranes. We will revisit the "E"xcellent antioxidants later.

Where do we find it?

✓ Green leafy vegetables
✓ Whole grains
✓ Nuts
✓ Vegetable oils
✓ Salmon
✓ Trout
✓ Cod
✓ Turnip greens

✓ Kiwis
✓ Avocado – Avocado is often known for its high content of healthy fats but did you know that just 1 cup (250 g) of mashed avocado contains over 20 different vitamins and minerals, including a high percentage of vitamin E? Avocados also contain anti-inflammatory phytosterols and antioxidants, zeaxanthin and lutein, important for brain health.

Not Enough Magnesium?

I would love to call this mineral, Magnificent Magnesium, taking into account the magnitude of its uses. Did you know that magnesium is involved in over 300 biochemical pathways in the human body? Remember MM — It's good for both: the mind and muscles.

We need magnesium to reduce anxiety, depression, restlessness, help us sleep, control blood sugar and blood pressure. It actually activates the enzymes required to produce serotonin and dopamine, helps you relax and has also been found to be beneficial in reducing muscle cramps, aches, and insomnia.

Where do we find it?

✓ Kale
✓ Spinach
✓ Broccoli
✓ Legumes
✓ Nuts
✓ Seeds
✓ White or navy beans
✓ Halibut
✓ Dark chocolate
✓ Brown rice

- ✓ Quinoa
- ✓ Black beans
- ✓ Edamame
- ✓ Tofu

Not Enough Selenium?

Selenium is known for its antioxidant properties as it helps make glutathione, which reduces inflammation in the brain. It also plays a role in regulating thyroid activity. Without selenium, we would feel tired and lethargic, irritable and prone to depression. Let's "Se"lebrate with selenium.

Where do we find it?

- ✓ Walnuts
- ✓ Liver
- ✓ Shrimp
- ✓ Brazil nuts
- ✓ Fish
- ✓ Garlic
- ✓ Whole grains
- ✓ Chicken
- ✓ Legumes
- ✓ Eggs
- ✓ Cottage cheese
- ✓ Brown rice
- ✓ Seeds
- ✓ Mushrooms
- ✓ Oats
- ✓ Spinach
- ✓ Bananas

Not Enough Zinc?

Let's get in sync with this potent mineral. Zinc helps us make vital proteins, regulate gene expression and DNA. We also need zinc to not only to make neurotransmitters but also ensure that our neurotransmitters function properly. Zinc is required for neurogenesis in the hippocampus in the brain and is important for memory. Researchers have found that sufficient amounts of zinc can reduce the time needed to fall asleep (sleep latency) and increase the quantity and quality of sleep.

Lack of motivation, loss of appetite, depression, poor memory, and even hyperactivity are symptoms of zinc deficiency. Bottom line: not enough zinc is implicated in a variety of mental health problems, so think about zinc.

Where do we find it?

✓ Beef
✓ Chicken
✓ Fish and shellfish
✓ Legumes
✓ Whole grains
✓ Pork
✓ Cashews
✓ Oysters

Not Enough Iron?

If you find yourself feeling tired and lethargic with a lack of energy to do exercise, also having symptoms of depression, irritability, brain fog, zero motivation, and appetite, there's a good chance that your iron levels are low. We need iron to make amino acids, collagen (discussed later), neurotransmitters and hormones.

Where do we find it?

- ✓ Red meat
- ✓ Eggs
- ✓ Fruit
- ✓ Green leafy vegetables
- ✓ Beans
- ✓ Asparagus
- ✓ Liver
- ✓ Lamb
- ✓ Oysters
- ✓ White beans
- ✓ Beef
- ✓ Tofu
- ✓ Lentils
- ✓ Quinoa
- ✓ Fortified cereals
- ✓ Brown rice
- ✓ Oats
- ✓ Pumpkin
- ✓ Squash
- ✓ Nuts and seeds

Some points to "iron" out — foods rich in vitamin C enhance iron absorption so best take iron with vitamin C. Iron absorption is decreased with some blood pressure medication, calcium, and antacids. Methylxanthines and tannins from tea can also decrease the absorption of iron, so if you're a tea drinker, be mindful to have your tea at least half an hour before taking iron.

Not Enough Iodine?

There we go again, what we put in is what we get out. Without this mineral, we would feel tired and lethargic with low mood as it plays a vital role in the functioning of our thyroid gland, nerves, and muscles.

Where do we find it?

- ✓ Cod
- ✓ Shrimp
- ✓ Tuna
- ✓ Iodized salt
- ✓ Eggs

Not Enough Chromium?

Remember the blood sugar spikes, mentioned earlier, that we need to avoid? The peaks and valleys of emotions, as a result of blood sugar imbalances, can be controlled with the help of chromium as it improves the functioning of insulin and helps control blood sugars. Chromium is also needed to make the neurotransmitter acetylcholine for nerve and brain activities that control memory and muscle energy.

Where do we get it?

- ✓ Meat
- ✓ Poultry
- ✓ Fish
- ✓ Nuts
- ✓ Eggs
- ✓ Brussel sprouts
- ✓ Broccoli
- ✓ Mushrooms
- ✓ Oats
- ✓ Asparagus

Not enough neurotransmitters? Here is how you would feel without the right balance of neurotransmitters, and what to eat to produce them (list below adapted from nutrition expert and author, Patrick Holford, 2003).

Not Enough Neurotransmitter Acetylcholine?

Here's what you would experience:

- Deterioration of memory and imagination
- Fewer dreams
- Increased confusion
- Forgetfulness and disorganization
- Mental exhaustion
- Poor concentration
- Difficulty learning new things

What to eat:

Foods rich in the nutrient called choline, which help build acetylcholine.

- ✓ Organic/free-range eggs
- ✓ Organic or wild fish – especially salmon, mackerel, sardines. Be mindful of the mercury content in fish as high levels of mercury can build up over time and damage the brain. The good news is that most fish are low in mercury (salmon, hake, herring, haddock, mullet, char, sole, mackerel, Pollock, sardines, trout, shellfish, canned "light" tuna such as skipjack, tongol and yellowfin). Larger fish have lived longer and have the highest levels of mercury. To avoid getting 'caught in the mercury net', limit the main

culprits such as; canned albacore (white) tuna, shark, swordfish, marlin and escolar.

- ✓ Organ meats
- ✓ Chicken
- ✓ Shrimp

Avoid:

- Sugar
- Deep-fried food and junk foods
- Refined and processed foods
- Alcohol

Not Enough Neurotransmitter Serotonin?

Here's what you would experience:

- Low mood
- Difficulty sleeping
- Feeling disconnected
- Lacking joy
- Anxiety
- Aggression
- Alcohol or drug abuse
- Cravings especially for sweet foods

What to eat:

Foods rich in tryptophan, which help produce serotonin.

- ✓ Fish
- ✓ Fruit
- ✓ Eggs

✓ Avocado
✓ Low-fat cheese
✓ Lean organic poultry
✓ Tofu
✓ Liver
✓ Walnuts
✓ Flaxseeds
✓ Pumpkin seeds
✓ Almonds
✓ Bananas
✓ Plums
✓ Tomatoes
✓ Legumes
✓ Broccoli

5-HTP at a dose of 100–300 mg has been shown to give good results promoting and maintaining sleep and helping with depression as it converts to serotonin and melatonin. Serotonin helps keep you emotionally balanced. Check with your physician or registered dietitian before trying out any supplements.

Avoid:

• Alcohol

Not Enough Neurotransmitter Dopamine?

Here's what you would experience:

• Lack of drive and motivation
• Lack of enthusiasm
• Crave stimulants and sugar
• Depression

- Boredom
- Mental and physical fatigue, regardless of how well you sleep
- Lack of focus and concentration
- Trouble waking up in the morning
- Low sex drive

What to eat:

Foods rich in tyrosine, which produce dopamine:

- ✓ Fruit and vegetables high in vitamin C
- ✓ Blueberries
- ✓ Walnuts
- ✓ Chia seeds
- ✓ Hemp seeds
- ✓ Grass-fed beef and lamb
- ✓ Kale
- ✓ Collards
- ✓ Brussel sprouts
- ✓ Chard
- ✓ Cabbage
- ✓ Salmon
- ✓ Mackerel
- ✓ Dark chocolate >70 % cacao
- ✓ Almonds

Have regular, small, frequent balanced meals. Deficiencies of vitamin B6, magnesium, iron, vitamin C, vitamin D, and vitamin B3 can alter dopamine levels. Dive back to the previously mentioned food sources of these powerful nutrients covered earlier.

Avoid:

    ✓ Caffeinated drinks and medication or supplements containing caffeine

Not Enough Neurotransmitter GABA?

Here's what you would experience:

- Difficulty relaxing
- Can't switch off
- Anxious about things
- Irritable
- Being self-critical

What to eat:

    ✓ Dark green leafy vegetables
    ✓ Nuts and seeds
    ✓ Bananas
    ✓ Eggs
    ✓ Brown rice
    ✓ Halibut
    ✓ Mackerel
    ✓ Fermented foods such as Kefir (more of this in next chapter)
    ✓ Oolong tea
    ✓ Shrimp
    ✓ Berries
    ✓ Citrus fruit

Avoid:

- Sugar
- Alcohol
- Caffeinated drinks

I am sure you have noticed that alcohol appears quite frequently on most of the lists of what to avoid. Alcohol is another culprit and here's why.

Earlier on, I mentioned vitamin B1 is easily depleted with excessive alcohol consumption, which can often lead to a condition called Wernicke-Korsakoff syndrome giving one symptoms of depression, anxiety, confusion, and loss of memory. It's a no-brainer that excessive alcohol can damage the brain and deplete nutrients. The more alcohol one consumes, the more the need to replenish nutrients.

In terms of how we feel, alcohol works mainly on the neurotransmitter GABA, which rises after a drink, but as the drink wears off GABA levels fall and grumpiness kicks in leaving one feeling moody, irritable and craving for another drink.

The next day, there's the down-regulation we mentioned earlier. The brain down-regulates after the influx of GABA and the pleasure-reward seeking neurotransmitter dopamine from the night before. In this down-regulation mode, the levels of our good feeling neurotransmitters are low and we would actually feel? Yes, you guessed it, DOWN.

After excessive drinking, there goes the mood, drive, motivation, pleasure, sleep, energy levels and ability to connect.

Be mindful of these feelings, and try to catch them before they catch you in their web of negativity. Pull yourself out of it quickly by staying positive, doing activities to sprout your neurons and, very importantly, feeding your brain with the right nutrients it needs to help you think clearly and elevate your mood. Even if your appetite is affected and you're in no mood to eat, get those brain-boosting blueberries and vital nutrients in your system somehow, even if in supplemental form, to help you bounce back. When those feelings of anxiety start brewing, make sure you're eating small, frequent, fibre-containing meals to keep those blood sugars stable. Urges and cravings come in waves. Ride the surge, and it will pass. Say "Cheers to moderation," and "Three cheers to healthy eating"— it is the definitely the way to go.

On an empowering note, remember neurogenesis in Chapter 1? According to an article written by Dr. Josh Axe, physician of natural medicine and clinical nutritionist, "Hippocampal neurogenesis is resilient and has been shown to recover following 30 days of abstinence from alcohol."

Exposure to toxins, smoke or other pollutants, generate free radicals, which are highly reactive unpaired electrons that can cause damage in the body. Free radicals can also be produced in the body during metabolic processes and can cause oxidative damage to the brain. That's where antioxidants are protective. According to Harvard publications, "antioxidant" is a general term for any compound that can counteract free radicals, which damage DNA, cell membranes and other parts of cells. Antioxidants prevent oxidative stress, which appear to be a common thread in various neurological and emotional conditions such as Alzheimer's disease, anxiety disorders, ADHD, dementia, and depression.

Where do we get antioxidants from?

- ✓ Vitamin C, E mentioned earlier
- ✓ Selenium
- ✓ Flavonoids and anthocyanins found in blueberries and onions. Research shows that consuming flavonoids leads to significant improvement in blood flow to the brain.

✓ Catechins, found in green tea
✓ Carotenoids such as lutein found in kale and plums and lycopene found in tomatoes
✓ Hesperetin found in oranges and other citrus fruit
✓ Grapeseed extract – rich in proanthocyanidins that protect cells against antioxidant damage. Grape seed polyphenols support healthy circulation to the brain by enhancing tone, elasticity, and strength of capillaries and other blood vessels. According to Shi et al. (2003), scientific studies have shown that the antioxidant power of proanthocyanidins is 20 times greater than vitamin E and 50 times greater than vitamin C.

Take-away messages of this chapter: Empower yourself to recharge, reboot, rejuvenate and elevate by conquering the culprits. A great thought to be mindful of is: be aware of not only what you eat but also of what you don't eat. Vitamin and mineral deficiencies are preventable and having enough of the good stuff in your diet can improve your memory, sharpen your mind, increase your energy and vitality and give you a greater overall sense of well-being. Lovely quote, by Jean Anthelme Brillat-Savarin, author of *The Physiology of Taste*, "Tell me what you eat, and I will tell you who you are."

CHAPTER 5

Healthy Gut, Healthy Brain?
Let's Get Brainy About Our Gut

Did you know that the gut is now being regarded as "the second brain." Yes. Say hello to brain number 2. Its true, not just a "gut feeling." Just like the brain, the gut is also found to produce those feel-good neurotransmitters dopamine and GABA and guess what? About 95 % of our serotonin, responsible for our happy feelings, is actually produced in the gut.

The gut-brain connection is fascinating and research in this area is continuously exploding, exploring the bi-directional communication that occurs via the gut and the brain (the gut-brain axis). Bottom line — the gut and brain share an intimate relationship where the gut affects the brain and the brain affects the gut via the vagus nerve (the only cranial nerve that passes from the skull all the way to the gut).

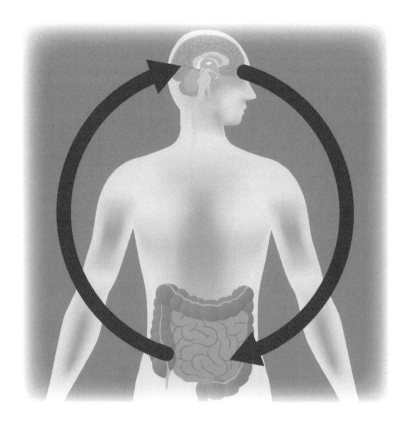

So, how does food fit into this equation?

In the previous chapter, I mentioned that what you eat, and the ecosystem of your gut will determine how your gut will function. We need our gut to function well for us to feel well. Also, remember neuroplasticity (the brain's ability to restructure and repair itself) from Chapter 1? Well, our gut also plays a vital role in creating BDNF required to produce new brain cells.

When we eat unhealthily, have poor digestion or an improper balance of bacteria in the gut, we can negatively impact our brain. Signals from the gut to the brain can be inflammatory in nature. Our body is meant to have an inflammatory response as a survival mechanism to protect itself from infection and injury. This is natural as long as it's not long lasting. If inflammation is prolonged in the gut, for example, from certain foods we eat, this inflammation in the gut may actually cause inflammation in the brain, affecting the production of our feel-good neurotransmitters and altering our thoughts and feelings.

Bacteria in our gut is one of the reasons research around the gut-brain connection is rocketing. Look out for the word gut **microbiome,** and watch it soon trumpet the airwaves because the bacteria in our gut have something to say.

So, what is the microbiome? It's a fancy word referring to the 100 trillion or so bacteria and microorganisms that live in your digestive tract. We have both good bacteria and bad bacteria in our gut, and we need to keep them in healthy balance.

One of the ways to keep our microbiome healthy is by eating healthily. Researchers are beginning to link the good bacteria in our gut to how we feel. We call the good bacteria **probiotics.** Probiotics have now become a popular inclusion in many diets, so the bad bacteria don't take over.

Dysbiosis is the term used to describe the disrupted balance of bacteria. We can avoid dysbiosis by making sure we have enough of the good bugs to keep the harmful bugs in check.

You would have seen the words *live cultures* on products while grocery shopping — on yogurt maybe? These live cultures refer to probiotics. We have always known that the strains of bacteria, Lactobacillus acidophilus and Bifidobacterium bifidum are good for digestion. Now, researchers are discovering many more strains of beneficial bacteria and exploring their role in mental health.

If we alter gut bacteria, we could alter our mood, handle stress better and reduce anxiety, as some strains of bacteria have been found to produce our feel-good neurotransmitters GABA, serotonin, and acetylcholine. These mind-altering probiotics are now termed **psychobiotics** as they regulate mood and brain function. It is said that good bacteria in our gut produce benzodiazapine-like substances, which are natural anti-anxiety neurochemicals.

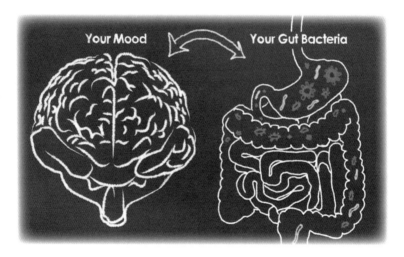

According to Kathleen Jade, naturopathic physician:

> Chronically elevated levels of inflammation throughout the body and brain are known to be one of the major underlying causes of depression and other mood and cognitive disorders. Some probiotics may have their effects in the brain by lowering inflammation.

Let's psych ourselves up with some probiotic lingo and what these probiotics have been linked to. Bear with me here — these names do sound like dinosaurs from *Jurassic Park*, but they are quite the opposite. Little bugs with big names, park in our gut and do a fair bit to help our brains. Let's do a quick drive by our park and get familiar with some of the beneficial bacteria strains.

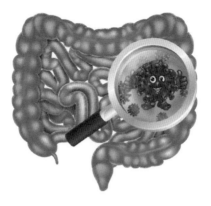

Probiotics include:

- Lactobacillus acidophillis
- Bifidobacterium bifidum
- Lactobacillus casei
- Bifidobacterium longum
- Lactobacillus helveticus
- Lactobacillus plantarium
- Lactobacillus bulgaricus

How was that drive by our park? Powered through those long names of our microscopic friends. But what do these names mean, and how have they been linked to how we feel? Let's take a look at the research; they are definitely worth the attention.

In a randomized, double-blind, placebo controlled clinical trial, published in *Nutrition Journal*, Ghodarz and his colleagues investigated the effects of probiotics on 40 patients a with major depressive disorder. After eight weeks, patients who received strains of Lactobacillus acidophilus, Lactobacillus casei, and Bifidobacterium bifidum, had beneficial effects on depression scores, insulin metabolism, reduced inflammation and an increase in the antioxidant glutathione.

In another double-blind, placebo controlled, randomized trial, published in *British Journal of Nutrition* by Messaoudi et al., probiotics Lactobacillus helveticus and Bifidobacterium longum, were found to be beneficial in reducing anxiety, stress, depression and anger hostility when taken for thirty days.

There's many, but let's go through just a few more studies. In an article published in *Beneficial Microbes Journal*, Kato-Kataoka and colleagues studied the effects of a fermented milk drink (kefir) containing Lactobacillus casei strain Shirota on medical students symptoms of psychological, physiological and physical stress. In this double-blind placebo controlled trial, medical students who consumed the fermented milk once a day for eight weeks showed reduced levels of stress and anxiety and increased levels of serotonin.

An animal study published in *Neuroscience Journal* by Liang, S. et al. found that the probiotic Lactobacilus Helveticus worked better than citalopram (an antidepressant) and lowered the stress hormone cortisol, restoring serotonin while reducing stress and anxiety.

According to Dr. Mike Dow, Bifidobacterium produces GABA; Streptococcus, Enterococcus, and Escherchia produce serotonin, and Lactobacillus produce both neurotransmitters acetylcholine and GABA. Lactobacillus plantarium has been linked to increasing feel-good dopamine and serotonin, reducing the stress hormone cortisol and helping with depression.

Overall, with results from studies above and many others out there, probiotics or psychobiotics have the potential to positively impact the brain, boost mood, alleviate depression and anxiety and reduce stress.

Probiotics also play a role in digestion and help us absorb nutrients. Besides reducing inflammation, they also help metabolism and influence the way we store fat.

The next time you see those dinosaur-sounding names written at the back of a probiotic supplement, you know what they mean and what they have been linked to. Speaking of probiotic supplements, be on the lookout for those containing at least 10 BILLION CFU (meaning centrifugal units) with a variety of different strains. The more variety the better as we want to diversify the bacteria in our gut.

Other than supplements, we can get probiotics from a variety of fermented foods such as:

- ✓ Kefir (one of the best sources with a variety of strains) — fermented drink, available in dairy or coconut
- ✓ Yogurt containing live cultures — remember the sugar labels, though. Avoid varieties with sugar, chemical preservatives, and artificial sweeteners as they disrupt the balance of good bacteria in the gut. Try *Skyr, an Icelandic cultured product* — it tastes delicious and creamy without the extra calories and sugar. Combine with blueberries, and it's like a guilt-free high protein dessert.
- ✓ Kimchi – a spicy Korean pickle made from cabbage or cucumber. Also a good source of vitamins and minerals.
- ✓ Sauerkraut – a fermented cabbage. Also contains choline used to make the neurotransmitter acetylcholine, mentioned earlier.
- ✓ Some pickles – keep in mind, though, that pickles stored in vinegar will not have probiotics as they are not naturally fermented with live cultures.
- ✓ Kombucha tea – this is a fermented black tea. It does contain probiotics but a small amount.
- ✓ Tempeh – fermented soy beans
- ✓ Buttermilk
- ✓ Dark chocolate
- ✓ Miso soup

✓ Natto – A traditional Japanese dish consisting of fermented soybeans

Did you know that stress and lack of sleep, raises cortisol levels and disrupt the good bacteria in the gut? So, there's another reason to start moving as exercise promotes a healthy balance of bacteria and can help us fight against stress and enhance sleep.

Some antibiotics also kill good bacteria, causing dysbiosis. Non-steroidal anti-inflammatory medication (aspirins, ibuprofens), create an imbalance in gut bacteria. Medications like proton-pump inhibitors that are used to treat acid reflux, gastritis, and ulcers, reduce acid in the stomach, and this could alter digestion leading to abdominal discomfort, bloating and mental fog.

So, we heard about PRObiotics. There's also PREbiotics. This is a term given to foods that are non-digestible and that feed the good bacteria in our gut, promoting their growth.

Examples of prebiotics are:

✓ Garlic
✓ Onions
✓ Leeks
✓ Artichoke
✓ Yams
✓ Chickory
✓ Legumes
✓ Oatmeal
✓ Bananas
✓ Asparagus

Prebiotics also reduce inflammation and lower insulin resistance. Remember the glycation process I mentioned in the previous chapter where glucose binds to proteins triggering inflammation? Prebiotics help reduce this.

5.1 Leaky gut? Leaky brain?

Let's "leak" out this information. After eating a meal, the lining of our intestine decides what gets absorbed into the bloodstream. If the lining is working well, it forms a tight barrier giving us better control of what we send into our blood. We all have a bit of a leaky gut, and that's how it's supposed to be, but when the gut lining is unhealthy, there are bigger holes or gaps in the lining and partially digested food or bad bacteria can pass through to the bloodstream.

Poor absorption of nutrients can lead to fatigue, bloating and inflammation in the gut, which as we discussed earlier, can alter our thinking, lead to depression and other mood disorders.

Omega-3 fats are known for their anti-inflammatory effects. In an article from *Surgical Neurology,* by Maroon and Bost (2006), controlled studies found that omega-3 fatty acids from fish oil had an equivalent effect, to non-steroidal anti-inflammatory medication such as ibuprofen, in reducing pain and inflammation and may appear to be a safer alternative.

We may think we are getting enough omega-3s via food (such as oily fish) or supplements, but what we really do need to think about is our omega-3 to omega-6 ratio, which needs to be 1:1. Unfortunately, many diets contain more omega-6 fats compared to omega-3 fats. Omega-6 fats (from processed vegetable oils such as soybean oil, corn oil, cottonseed oil, almond oil, flaxseed oil, safflower oil, sesame seed oil, and sunflower oil), have the opposite effect of omega-3s and are regarded as pro-inflammatory.

When we consume more omega-6s, omega-3 fats struggle to compete with omega-6s for enzymes in our cell membranes, and the result is exactly what we don't want — more inflammation.

When choosing meat and poultry, always opt for those that are grass-fed as they will have a higher level of omega-3 and less of the omega-6. Cattle that are grain-fed are often fed soy and corn, often genetically modified, which have a higher omega-6 content, promoting inflammation.

According to Dr. Caroline Leaf, in grass-fed cattle, the ratio of omega-3 to omega 6 is 1:1.53 and in grain-fed cattle, the ratio of omega-3 to omega-6 is 1:7.65. Stressed animals will have higher levels of stressed hormones and will increase inflammation, so it's best to choose free-range and organically raised meat and poultry, whenever possible.

A diet high in sugar, unhealthy trans fats, foods that are processed, additives, saturated fats, alcohol and low in fibre can cause inflammation and promote the growth of harmful bacteria, disrupting the balance of bacteria in the gut.

5.2 Collagen and the gut-brain? Are you clued up on collagen?

When we think of collagen, we think of hair, skin, joint health and wound healing. But did you know that this protein has a role in gut health and can actually aid in repairing the holes of our leaky gut, reducing inflammation?

Collagen provides the building blocks for healing. It is made up of a variety of amino acids, glycine being the dominant one and contributing to most of collagen's beneficial properties. Glycine and the amino acids glutamine and proline from collagen have been found to help repair the gut lining, healing a leaky gut.

The high glycine content of collagen also stimulates the production of stomach acid, improving the digestion of food. We know from earlier that better digestion and a healthier gut contribute to a healthier brain. Glycine is known to buffer the stress hormone cortisol and can, therefore, help calm us, relax us and improve our quality of sleep. Collagen helps give cohesion to tissues, keeping them flexible. Blood actually runs off of collagen as well, so without it, we would feel tired and lethargic, as blood carries energy.

There are over 20 types of collagen but the most commonly found types are:

+ Type 1
  -most abundant and present in over 90 % of tissues of all tendons, ligaments, bones, teeth, skin, arteries

+ Type 2
  -found in joints, cartilage and eyes

+ Type 3
  -forms a mesh around liver, lymph, bone marrow, lungs

+ Type 4
  -found in the respiratory tract, bronchial tubes, lungs, intestines, the heart and kidneys

+ Type 5
  -found in hair and cell surfaces

Collagen in our bodies depletes with age. After 20, we lose 1–2 % collagen a year, decreasing skin elasticity and causing hair and nails to become brittle. Replenishing collagen can improve skin elasticity, and

I have seen this protein work wonders healing wounds and pressure ulcers in many of my long-term care residents.

Where do we get it?

Bone broth is rich in collagen and high in glycine, proline, and hydroxyproline, which keep the lining of the gut wall smooth and protected.

Collagen is available in many other forms such as; marine collagen, bovine collagen from grass-fed cows, and collagen from chicken and pork. The best form of collagen is hydrolyzed collagen in peptide form as it most easily absorbed. It has been broken down by water making the amino acids shorter, requiring minimal digestion.

Dose: 10 g per day for maintenance but this may be increased depending on individualized nutritional requirements.

Keep in mind that we need vitamin C to metabolize collagen. When we have low stomach acid from medication that reduce acidity, we are not able to digest collagen and would also experience symptoms such as iron deficiency, vitamin B12 deficiency, and indigestion.

What depletes collagen?

- Sugar
- Alcohol
- Smoking

This chapter covered yet another powerful link between food and the mind via the gut-brain connection. Brain chemistry can be altered by manipulating the bacteria in our gut and keeping them in balance. Be mindful to avoid foods that cause inflammation and choose to protect your gut. Nourish your gut microbiome to nourish your brain, and you will also have a restful sleep.

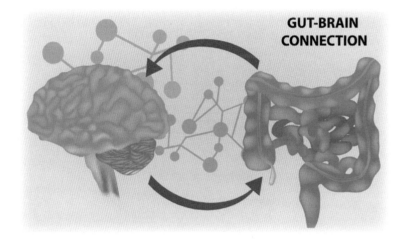

CHAPTER 6

Eat Well, Think Well,
Feel Well and Improve Your Memory

6.1 It's all "in the mind"

Have you ever noticed the number of diet books on the shelves of bookstores? What about the countless articles on new fad diets popping up on the internet? Wow, there's tons of information out there and so many different diets to follow. I often see patients in my practice who have tried every diet there is and find themselves caught up in a dietary mess, confused and in urgent need of an individualized nutrition approach to eating for their specific health goals. There is really so much conflicting nutrition jargon out there, and it can become quite overwhelming at times.

Diets that have achieved great results, and what many experts recommend as the healthiest, include the Mediterranean Diet and the DASH Diet. You would have likely come across the Mediterranean Diet, which is very popular for years now and the DASH diet, which stands for Dietary Approaches to Stop Hypertension. These diets have been well-known to be protective against cardiovascular conditions like heart attacks, high blood pressure, stroke, and diabetes.

This book is about the link between food and the mind and when it comes to brain health and memory, it is really all in the MIND. The MIND diet focuses on improving brain function, memory and preventing Alzheimer's disease and is, actually, a mashup of the Mediterranean and DASH diet. This combination is a great dietary approach to eating for brain health that's easy to follow.

MIND stands for the Mediterranean-DASH Intervention for Neurodegenerative Delay. Studies done by nutritional epidemiologist Dr. Martha Clare Morris and her colleagues at Rush University Medical Centre found that the MIND diet lowered the risk of Alzheimer's disease by 53 % if followed rigorously, and 35 % when followed moderately.

Researchers also found that the longer a person followed the MIND diet, the lower the risk of developing Alzheimer's disease. The Mediterranean Diet also lowered Alzheimer's risk by 54 % and the DASH diet by 39 %.

The MIND diet is low in high-fat foods and is mainly plant-based, focusing particularly on eating foods such as green leafy vegetables and berries, the healthy foods for the brain. These foods possibly reduce oxidative stress from free radicals (mentioned earlier) and prevent inflammation. Participants who ate one to two servings of green vegetables a day had a "dramatic decrease in the rate of cognitive decline compared to people who ate fewer greens. It was about the equivalent of being 11 years younger in age," said Dr. Morris.

The MIND diet focuses on two categories: ten foods good for brain health and five food categories that are unhealthy for the brain and should be avoided.

Let's get mindful of these brainy foods:

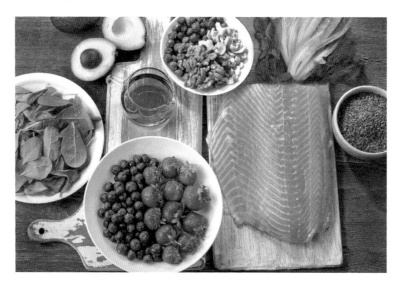

1) Live well with *leafy greens*

- ✓ Go for green as much as you can. Try to have at least 6 servings per week.
- ✓ When it comes to cooked vegetables, for example, cooked kale or spinach; ½ cup = 1 serving.
- ✓ If you're having salads, 1 cup of raw vegetables = 1 serving.
- ✓ Green leafy veggies, in particular, are extra special in offering protection to the brain and have been found to reduce the rate of cognitive decline. They also contain folic acid, lutein and other nutrients that can help preserve brain function.
- ✓ Leafy greens also improve oxygen transport throughout the body, help decrease harmful inflammation and increase red blood cell production.

✓ Another benefit – leafy greens add healthy fibre to your diet, and we know from earlier chapters – we love fibre.

✓ Green leafy veggies get a "green light" for sure. Green means "go". So, go ahead and load up on:

   ➤ Spinach
   ➤ Kale
   ➤ Swiss chard
   ➤ Beet greens
   ➤ Collards
   ➤ Broccoli
   ➤ Arugula
   ➤ Romaine lettuce

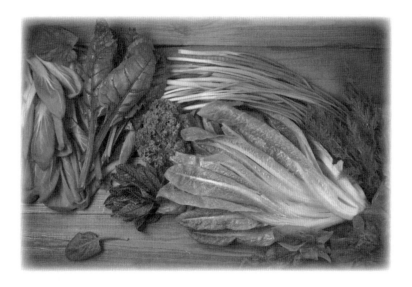

2) Create colour with ***other vegetables***

- ✓ Include 1 serving of other vegetables daily, preferably non-starchy vegetables, so you're getting the nutrients without the additional calories.
- ✓ Again here, 1 serving is 1 cup of raw vegetables or ½ cup of cooked vegetables.
- ✓ Include other green, orange, yellow, red, purple, and white vegetables. The goal here is a variety of protective phytochemicals, and we want many of them for our brain. The more colour, the better.

- ✓ Let's "vegetate" towards:

- ➤ Asparagus
- ➤ Green beans
- ➤ Green peppers
- ➤ Carrots
- ➤ Butternut
- ➤ Squash
- ➤ Yellow peppers
- ➤ Red peppers
- ➤ Tomato
- ➤ Beets
- ➤ Eggplant
- ➤ Purple cabbage
- ➤ Onions
- ➤ Garlic
- ➤ Cauliflower
- ➤ Mushrooms

3) The ***berry*** bunch, our brain's best fruit friends

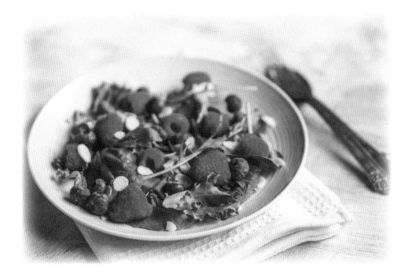

✓ Try to have at least 2 or more servings a week of brain-loving berries.

✓ 1 serving of berries = ½ cup

✓ Blueberries and strawberries are especially powerful in protecting the brain as they contain powerful polyphenols and phytochemicals that protect brain cells by fighting free radical damage, reducing inflammation and removing toxic proteins that occur with age.

✓ Other diets focus on having fruit in general, but in terms of the brain, berries are definitely the way to go.

✓ Research has been done on strawberries and blueberries, although raspberries and blackberries can also be included as they are high in similar antioxidants.

4) Go a little ***nuts*** now and then

  ✓ It's OK to get nutty with 1 serving of nuts daily, which equates to 1 ounce or ¼ cup.
  ✓ Walnuts are winning in the nut department. Research indicates that eating more walnuts can help improve memory, concentration, and brain processing speeds.
  ✓ They also have polyphenols and omega-3s, which help reduce inflammation.
  ✓ Watch the calories, though — nuts contribute significant calories, so be mindful of your portions or you will pack on the pounds.

5) Love those LOW GI ***legumes***

  ✓ Remember LOW GI foods from Chapter 4. We want to choose them more often because they cause a slower more gradual release of fuel to the brain and contain fibre with numerous benefits.
  ✓ Lentils and beans such as kidney beans, pinto beans, black beans, and chickpeas are great varieties to choose from.
  ✓ We can have 3–4 servings per week.
  ✓ 1 serving is ½ cup cooked legumes

6) ***Whole grains*** for blood flow to the brain

  ✓ Whole grains promote a healthy cardiovascular system.
  ✓ Foods that promote a healthy cardiovascular system are also good for the brain because if there is poor circulation of blood to the brain, your memory and thinking may be impaired.

✓ 3 servings per day with 1 wholegrain serving = 1 slice whole grain bread, ½ cup cooked brown rice, quinoa, whole grain pasta, oatmeal, 1 cup 100 % whole grain, ready-to-eat breakfast cereal.

7) Catch of the day, oily *fish*

✓ Oily fish such as salmon, trout, sardines, herring, and mackerel have DHA, an omega-3 essential for brain function.

✓ A higher intake of DHA is thought to delay brain aging and improve memory and thinking skills. It may also help prevent the buildup of protein plaques in the brain, called beta-amyloid plaques (as seen in Alzheimer's disease) and reduce inflammation.

✓ 1 or more servings per week is ideal.

✓ 1 serving of fish is about 3 ounces (90 g) cooked.

✓ Go feast on fish!

8) Pop in some *poultry*

✓ 2 servings per week

✓ 1 serving of chicken or turkey = 3 ounces (90 g) cooked

✓ Chicken and turkey, and having less red meat, are associated with a lower risk of Alzheimer's disease.

✓ Remember to choose grass-fed, organic, free-range varieties, as mentioned previously.

✓ Avoid deep-frying, battered or crumbed varieties

9) Oil up with **olive oil**

   ✓ Olive oil should be your primary oil. It is a rich source of monounsaturated fat, the type that reduces inflammation and keeps blood vessels working properly. Extra virgin olive oil contains oleocanthal, a protective phytochemical that may boost production of two key enzymes believed to be critical in removing the beta-amyloid protein plaques from the brain, again as seen in Alzheimer's disease.

10) Just a little **wine** is fine

   ✓ Not too much though, 1 glass per day equal to 5 ounces (150 ml)
   ✓ Studies suggest that one glass of wine per day helps preserve memory and reduce Alzheimer's risk.
   ✓ Low levels of alcohol are thought to have anti-inflammatory effects on the brain. Too much alcohol, however, can damage the brain. Don't forget to watch the sugar and calories as it can also easily lead to weight gain.

Foods in battle with the brain, in other words, *try to avoid:*

1) Red meats: eat rarely
2) Butter/margarine: A maximum of 1 tablespoon per day. Stick to the olive oil. You could try avocado oil as well.
3) Cheese: One serving or less per week.
4) Pastries and sweets – as yummy as they may be, avoid processed or junk foods, and commercially prepared baked goods. Many contain trans fats, which are extremely harmful and known to cause many diseases from heart disease to Alzheimer's disease.
5) Fried or fast food – less than one serving per week or avoid completely.

A quick glance at the research — in a randomized, controlled study published in the *Archives of Neurology*, Dr. Craft and her colleagues found that participants in the study who followed a Western diet high in saturated fat and sugar for a month, had increased inflammation and levels of beta-amyloid protein buildup, playing a role in the development of Alzheimer's disease compared to participants following a more heart-healthy diet with the same number of calories.

Even if you're unable to follow the MIND diet strictly consuming all the servings, don't give up. Continue to follow it, even moderately as research indicates that even following it moderately can give you benefits. The MIND diet is relatively new but observational studies indicate promising results and research is evolving in this area.

6.2 Let's go with the "flow"

Ever experienced a state of flow? Maybe you have and didn't realize it or maybe you haven't but if you're set on reaching a goal to complete a task, it's a great and fascinating space to be absorbed in.

If you find yourself lost in a profound state of concentration while performing a task and at the same time being able to disconnect completely from your thoughts, keeping intense focus without having to really think, then congratulations, you have reached a peak performance state of mind and going with the flow.

According to an article published in *Conscious Cognition*, Gyurcovics et al. describe "flow" as a special mental state characterized by deep concentration that occurs during the performance of optimally challenging tasks.

Steven Kotler, director of The Flow Genome Project, says:

> In flow, every action, every decision, arises seamlessly from the last. We are so focused on the task at hand that all else falls away. Action and awareness merge. Our sense of self vanishes. Our sense of time distorts and performance goes through the roof.

Remember in Chapter 2, we learned how to, "**Stop Those Thoughts — STT.**" In a flow state, you are able to complete a task, almost on autopilot without any of those negative thoughts interfering. In fact, you complete your task or project so efficiently with your skills, to the point of losing track of time.

The analytical part of the brain shuts down and creativity explodes on another level, and there you go, with the flow, and you are able to write an entire chapter, swim all those laps, paint that wonderful picture or design something extraordinary.

> In a study by Marino Bonaiuto et al., flow is a psychological state encompassed by "energized concentration, optimal enjoyment, full involvement (in a task), motivation and intrinsic interest."

So, how do we explain this high functioning, stress-free, calming state of mind, where there is clarity of thought with great ideas, allowing creativity to flourish?

We learned all about our neurotransmitters in previous chapters and how drastically they contribute to how we feel. Our performance is also affected. In a flow state, there is an increase in blood flow to the brain, and our feel-good neurotransmitters are released. There is a release of norepinephrine and dopamine (which enhance drive, motivation and focus), endorphins (which block pain, enabling us to burn the midnight oil with ease), serotonin (the happy feeling neurotransmitter giving us enjoyment during the task) as well as anandamide (helping us think outside the box). With these five rewarding neurotransmitters released simultaneously, flow state can become pleasurable, productive and possibly addictive.

Scientists have created a term called "the flow channel", where flow is known to occur — at the half-way point between the feelings of boredom and anxiety. A task must not be too difficult to allow fear or negative thoughts to set in (**STT, remember**) and at the same time the task must not be too simple, or we begin to lose interest.

According to Steven Kotler, as a rule of thumb, "The challenge must be 4 % greater than the skills." An overachiever would fly over 4 % aiming for difficult tasks and get overwhelmed with burn out, missing the peaceful, productive, pleasurable state of flow. Underachievers miss the 4 % point because at this point the task begins to feel a little more out of their comfort zone, and they fall back without reaching the meaningful, motivational flow state.

As with anything you're working on, whether it's a project or task or healthy eating, start slowly, step by step. Progress takes time, so give yourself some time to get into the flow of things. Diving into a fanatical frenzy to achieve rapid results may leave you feeling exhausted. Know that it doesn't have to be that way. Step out of your comfort zone gradually, and you will find a happy medium that works wonderfully for you.

If you need help to achieve a flow state and enhance brain function, here are a few natural ways to do so, using *nootropics*. Nootropics are substances that can be taken to improve mental performance, boost memory, focus, creativity, and motivation. There are many varieties but best to stick to the natural options.

Let's flow through a few:

1) L-Theanine

- This is an ingredient or naturally occurring amino acid, derived from green tea, which is enhanced when combined with caffeine.
- It has been known for its calming effects on the brain by reducing beta brainwaves, which are associated with nervousness, anxiety, and hyperactivity.
- It stimulates alpha brainwaves keeping us alert and focused while at the same time keeping us calm and relaxed.
- L-Theanine has been used for centuries to induce relaxation for flow during meditation and is now used to help alleviate stress, enhance quality of sleep and improve mental focus.
- Dose: 100–200 mg, 1 to 3 times per day. (This may vary depending on the individual. Speak to your dietitian or qualified health care professional prior to taking any supplements.)

2) Phosphatidyl Serine (PS)

- This is a phospholipid (or fat) that forms the myelin sheath (the insulating layer around nerves) and helps to make neurotransmitters acetylcholine, norepinephrine, dopamine and serotonin, enhancing mood and mental ability.
- PS has been found to improve memory, concentration, and learning.
- Researchers found an improvement in depressive symptoms after 30 days of PS. It may also protect cells from oxidative stress and decrease anxiety and hyperactivity.
- According to Dr. Thomas Crook, internationally recognized memory expert, PS can slow, halt, or reverse the decline of

memory and mental function due to aging. Dr. Crook and his colleagues found, in a double-blind trial, that administering 300 mg of PS daily could restore up to 12 years' worth of lost mental function.

+ Dose: 100–300 mg daily. (This may vary depending on the individual. Speak to your dietitian or qualified health care professional prior to taking any supplements.)

3) Bacopa monnieri and Rhodiola rosea

+ These are herbal nootropics that may help improve focus and memory and has been found to increase feel-good neurotransmitters GABA and serotonin, improving mood. Rhodiola rosea may also help reduce mental fatigue and help one adapt to periods of high stress. (Speak to your dietitian or qualified health care professional prior to taking any supplements).

4) L-Tyrosine

+ Helps replenish depleted neurotransmitters, dopamine, norepinephrine and epinephrine and may increase focus, memory and motivation for flow state.
+ Studies on L-Tyrosine have shown it to be beneficial to enhance cognition, especially in stressful situations. (Speak to your dietitian or qualified health care professional prior to taking any supplements)

At the end of this chapter, let this take-away idea flow into your mind: eating healthily for the brain is not as tricky as brain science. It's actually very simple, easy to follow, and it can be sustained over a long time to create and filter into a healthy lifestyle. The healthier your brain, the easier your compliance to any healthy eating plan. It all starts with the mind. When your mind is healthy and clear, everything flows and with this flow, you can experience memorable states that can elevate you, calm you and energize you at the same time, in the most natural way. It is amazing! So, keep going, keep flowing!

CHAPTER 7

Hydrate to Feel Great

Drink up this chapter — really "soak" this information in, because a dehydrated brain does not work well to win. We all know how vital it is to stay hydrated for overall good health and well-being, but bear in mind that the brain, specifically, needs fluids to function at its best. With insufficient fluid, one can be prone to poor memory, headaches, and tiredness. You may find yourself feeling irritable, restless, confused and your performance and productivity may be affected.

We need a minimum of 1.5–2 litres of fluid a day; that's 6–8 glasses (250 ml each), and water is the most, guilt-free, calorie-free and quenching way to hydrate to feel great. We lose about 1.5 litres of water through the skin, gut, lungs, and kidneys in our body's attempt to flush out toxins. We need to replenish the water we lose, to avoid getting dehydrated. Don't wait for that thirsty moment because, guess what? When you're thirsty, you are already dehydrated.

According to an article by Riebl et al. featured in ACSM's *Health Fitness Journal*, even mild dehydration — a body water loss of 1–2 % can impair cognitive performance and was linked to poor concentration, short-term memory problems, moodiness, anxiety and increased reaction times.

We definitely need to prevent our dehydrated state of mind and reduce the risk of cognitive decline, especially as we get older.

Be careful not to overhydrate, though, unless you're exercising. More than 2 litres a day can exert a greater workload on the kidneys, and you may dilute essential electrolytes. Electrolytes such as sodium, potassium, and magnesium are important minerals with an electric charge. We need to keep these minerals balanced, so muscles and nerves function well and cells do not get dehydrated. Drinking water intermittently throughout the day is the best approach.

Although water is best, other fluids can also contribute to our 1.5–2 litre per daily fluid requirement. When it comes to fluids, try avoiding sugar-containing beverages and beverages that are artificially-sweetened. These will only cause you to gain weight, keep you craving more sugary drinks (mentioned in earlier chapter) and also disrupt the good bacteria in our gut.

When drinking water with a meal, have it 15 minutes before a meal or after, but not during the meal as water can dilute stomach acid, required for better digestion.

If your water needs a boost, try adding ginger, mint or a few slices of lemon to add some zest to it. Lemon water is a lovely way to hydrate and nourish.

Lemons contain vitamin C, an antioxidant offering protection from oxidative stress and help prevent fatigue. Lemon water also helps with digestion and flushing out toxins. It contains bioflavonoids, which help prevent inflammation and as well as citric acid, which, when metabolized in the body, creates an alkaline environment, which also reduces inflammation. So, there are many reasons to gulp some warm lemon water when you're up each morning.

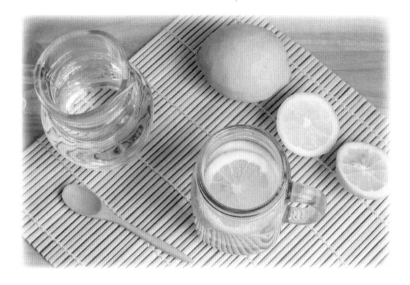

Teas are also great ways to get fluids. Black tea and green tea contain polyphenols that maintain the good bacteria in our gut. Organic ceremonial matcha tea is one of the most potent of the green tea varieties. Matcha is derived from the green tea leaves of the Camellia sinesis plant. The leaves are not steeped and discarded as with other green teas but are crushed into a fine powder and mixed into food and beverages. It is loaded with antioxidants and far more concentrated than other green teas. The darker the green, the more potent it is. It also contains EGCG mentioned earlier (an ingredient that can promote the growth of new brain cells) and L-Theanine, keeping us alert, focused and calm. Try ½ teaspoon in 6 oz (180 ml) water close to boiling but not quite or boiled water that has been allowed to stand for five minutes. It can also be added to smoothies, yogurt, stir-fry, and eggs.

Watch the caffeine, though. Matcha has more caffeine than steeped tea but less than coffee. Small amounts of caffeine are OK, but we don't want excessive amounts. The more caffeine you consume, the less sensitive your brain becomes to its own natural stimulants of dopamine and adrenalin.

You would then need more stimulants to feel normal and keep on pushing the body to produce more dopamine and adrenalin. You will eventually feel exhausted.

Tea, Coffee, Caffeine Run Down

Beverage	Quantity	Caffeine Content
Coffee – Instant	150 ml	40–105 mg
Espresso, Cappuccino, Latte		30–50 mg
Filter Coffee	150 ml	110–150 mg
Tea	150 ml	20–100 mg
Green Tea	150 ml	20–30 mg

Coffee contains three stimulants: caffeine, theobromine, and theophylline, all of which can disturb sleep patterns. Drinking three to four cups of coffee is OK in a day, but if you're concerned about the caffeine, decaffeinated options are great.

If you are a frequent coffee drinker and trying to cut down your coffee intake, try a cup of matcha green tea (mentioned earlier) before your first cup of coffee. You will notice that it's probably the only cup of coffee you will need in a day. Matcha tea gives a slow-releasing, more calming energy with no anxiety or crash, compared to the frequent crash and jittery feelings experienced after a cup of coffee wears off.

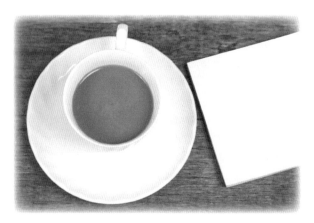

Energy drinks are often loaded with caffeine and sugar and should be avoided. Aim to have a glass of water after drinking coffee and two glasses of water after any alcoholic drink. "Drench" your mind with this thought: Did you know that fruit and vegetables also contain around 90 % of water? Two pieces of fruit and two servings of vegetables can provide 500 ml water.

End point of this quick chapter to "sip" in: if you're feeling moody, drink some water. During sleep, you haven't hydrated for about eight hours, so make sure you hydrate as soon as you rise. Drinking water makes us feel so refreshed that it can actually improve our state of mind.

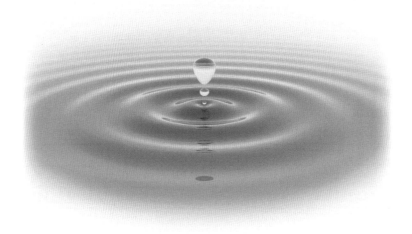

CHAPTER 8

Mindfully Moving to Wellness

To move to wellness, we have to move our minds. Let's start moving. Let's focus on YOU because YOU are the most important person in your life, and you deserve to become the best version of yourself. When you focus on yourself first, you put your best self forward, allowing all areas of your life to flourish.

Many of us have "go, go, go" schedules — we are on the move constantly, working long hours, skipping meals, driven by social media and racing against time. We often forget to practice any self-care or mindfulness during activities, especially during meal times.

In Chapter 5, we connected our minds to the gut-brain connection. It's a two-way street. Your mind can affect your digestion, and your digestion can affect your mind. Who would have thought that being stressed, angry or anxious while eating could actually affect your digestion? It's true. In our hectic lifestyles, when we do eventually get a chance to eat, we are often so preoccupied with thoughts of our stressful day or anxiously absorbed, contemplating what we have to do next, that we completely forget to eat mindfully and peacefully. We need to become aware of this and realize that we must quickly switch to positive thoughts to generate positive experiences. Letting go of the negative can be liberating.

When we have unhealthy stressful thoughts, unhealthy feelings emerge while eating. This negative state of mind can alter the way our food is digested and absorbed, causing inflammation, bloating or heartburn.

Be mindfully aware of your emotions and aim to be relaxed while eating.

The mind can play tricks on us — but with heightened awareness, we can actually play tricks to control our minds too.

Tune in to this bag of magical tricks:

- ✓ Don't eat on the go — you will notice that your mind hasn't registered that you've eaten and chances are that you're going to crave more food really soon. Take your time and eat slowly. By eating slowly, you will actually get full faster. If you gobble and go, you will miss the mind's sensation of satiety. It takes 20 minutes for your mind to register that you're full. If you eat too fast, you're definitely going to be eating more than you need to, when you were already full a while ago but didn't even realize it. That's the gut-brain connection again — it helps regulate appetite.
- ✓ Let your mind KNOW that you're eating. Drop out distractions like eating while watching television or reading while eating. Not only will you miss the enjoyment of devouring your delicious meal, but your mind will trick you into eating way more than you should, pushing you to grab more food later. When eating while watching TV becomes a habit, our minds generally associate these two activities with each other. Munch on this: it's all just an association of activities. This has

nothing to do with hunger, and you're basically setting yourself up to automatically reach for food every time you're watching TV or reading, without being aware of it. Another strong association to remember — when you go to the movies. On autopilot mode, we stand in line to order our sugary beverages and massive popcorn when we don't really need them. Try eating a healthy snack or meal prior to the movie. You can break these associations by being aware of these activities and behaviours and challenging your brain.

✓ When eating, savour every bite. Food has so much to offer — a healthy meal is like a beautiful picture. Take time in to enjoy the colours, flavours, and textures of every bite. Don't miss out on the deliciousness; your meal would feel much more satisfying, and you can drop the cravings later.

✓ Eat in the correct environment or the right setting. In other words, avoid eating at your desk at work, but if you do, be mindful of what you're eating instead of working and eating simultaneously. Put the brakes on eating in the car. Definitely a no-no. Make a deal with yourself to eat only in the correct setting: when you're seated comfortably and eating from a plate.

✓ Using a smaller plate will make your portions appear larger. Lovely way to control portions. I remember a patient of mine once said that he achieved excellent results in reaching his goal weight by eating in a smaller bowl. He managed his mind and weight and, in doing so, felt great.

✓ Clear the kitchen clutter. The more disorganized the kitchen, the more likely you will clutter your mind with cravings. Everything affects the mind, on some level. In an article by Vartanian et al. (2016) from the *Journal of Environment and Behavior*, it was found that women who had clutter in their kitchen were more stressed and took in twice as many calories.

✓ Be aware of visual cues. If you have unhealthy food available in your kitchen, when they are in your line of vision, you will be in the line of fire, with a burning desire to consume it. Keep healthy raw vegetable snacks at home, blueberries and a few walnuts. If you purchase unhealthy food items, you WILL eat it.

✓ Don't shop while hungry. You're going to buy all the snacks and delights you crave and may consume them as soon as you're home. If it's there, and you see it, chances are you will have it even when you don't need it, as mentioned in the previous point.

✓ Before you eat, ask yourself: Am I really hungry? How am I feeling? Am I angry, bored, sad? It is important to distinguish between emotional hunger cravings and physical hunger. An emotional hunger craving is usually suddenly onset and, chances are, you're not feeling great. Wait it out. Have a glass of water, and visit your questions in 15 minutes. Physical hunger develops over a longer duration and persists even after 15 minutes have passed. Be mindful and recognize emotional eating. Don't eat in an attempt to soothe anxiety, irritation or sadness. Be aware of the association between emotions and eating, and be mindful to **stop those thoughts (STT)** and BREAK THEM.

✓ When you're eating, try to stop when you're 75 % full, wait and re-evaluate: Am I still hungry? When you do this, in time you will realize you are no longer hungry after consuming 75 % of your meal and don't need to eat 100 % of it mindlessly.

So, we have "engorged" on a few strategies about being mindful of our behaviours, which can distract us from our path to wellness. We don't have to be overly fanatical about all this but simply aware, and it will slowly evolve into a greater and more meaningful practice later on.

If you give in to a craving at a party, while on holiday or while dining out, don't be so hard on yourself. Realize that there are about twenty-one main meals in a week, so if 1 meal does not go according to your plan, your brain will still reward you with an A+ grade of 95 %, so filter that into the equation. Forgive yourself with compassion and move on.

Always believe in yourself. Realize that progress takes time. If you're trying to lose weight, for example, and after a week, you have lost ½ kg — this may seem like a little, but taking into account we have fifty-two weeks a year, that's an impressive 26 kg for the year! So, keep going, and know that you have the power to create change and see progress, and if the plan doesn't work, tweak the plan, not the goal. You can make it happen.

We take care of numerous things in a day, but we often dismiss taking care of our minds. We all want to be happy and feel positive. We need to give ourselves a few minutes to be mindful while doing simple things, stop for a moment, breathe and take things in. Make time for yourself for what you may find relaxing — this could be anything from yoga, jogging in the park, doing a hike, golfing or cycling. Self-care does not have to be strenuous. Try reading, take a bubble bath, listen to your favourite songs, paint, create or treat yourself to a massage, try journaling.

Journaling is a fantastic, healthy practice, which will push you into action to make your dreams into a reality and keep you on your path to wellness. In doing so, you will master yourself, your mindsets, emotions, and behaviours. Journaling is known to reduce stress, manage depression and anxiety.

It also allows for motivational moments of self-talk and increases awareness and insight. So, write down your thoughts, what you ate, and how it made you feel. Keep writing. Write down the dreams and experiences you want to have and think of ideas to take you there, working towards them with gratitude. There is no such thing as failure — there are only growing experiences that help us build a foundation of achievement. Nothing is impossible. KNOW that your ideas matter and that you are important, capable, and deserving. Dedicate to learning and growing every day. Over the long term, your extraordinary mind will give you extraordinary results.

If you don't know how to start or what to write in your journal, start with a blank page, and at the top of it, in capital letters, write a note to yourself: MY TRUE PURPOSE IN LIFE FROM THIS DAY FORWARD IS TO BE THE BEST VERSION OF MYSELF. I AM GOING TO MAKE MYSELF SO PROUD. When we give ourselves love, care, and compassion, we can open our hearts in a way that can powerfully transform our lives. Believe in yourself, your experiences and talents, and do something that feeds your passion.

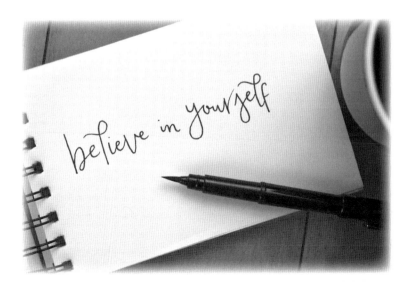

CONCLUSION

I hope that you have enjoyed reading this book as much as I enjoyed writing it, and I hope that at this point you're feeling uplifted and empowered and have fully digested the strong link between food and the mind. Dr. Gomez-Pinilla, professor of Neurosurgery and Psychological Science, who has analyzed more than 160 studies of foods effects on the brain, states in *Nature Reviews Neuroscience*, "Some foods are like pharmaceutical compounds; their effects are so profound, that the mental health of entire countries may be linked to them." This stresses the importance of becoming mindful of what we eat and how it makes us feel — We should really ask ourselves, "What will this food do for me, and how will it affect the way I feel afterwards?"

There is a ton of advice in the book about foods to increase neurogenesis, prevent deficiencies, improve memory and focus and nourish the brain. We are all special and unique with different health goals and needs. There is no one-size fits all approach. It is ideal to consult with a registered dietician to help work out a plan that's best suited to meet your individualized nutritional requirements, taking into account your patterns of eating, lifestyle, activity levels, health conditions, and medication. Intervention by a registered dietitian can lead to reduced nutrition-related side-effects of medication, improved cognition and mood, and enhanced well-being.

We need to give our bodies the right sustenance that delivers the right nutrients, to equip us with revitalizing energy, enabling us to push forward, to grow our potential and follow our dreams. Let *The Empowered Mind Diet Equation – Your Empowered Mind + Brain Healthy Diet* be the driving force behind your wellness and success. I wish you all the best in your journey to become the best version of yourself.

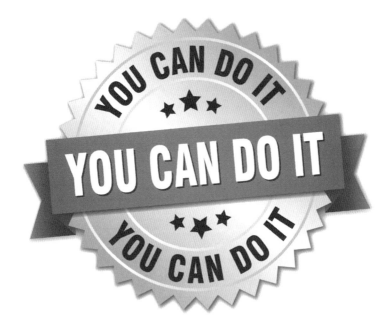

ACKNOWLEDGEMENTS

I loved writing this book. I especially enjoyed experiencing the process of sparking an idea, forming keywords scattered on a page, soon sprouting sentences, which would merge to form paragraphs, flowing to fill up a page and, thereafter, chapter by chapter — with lots of motivation, dedication and consistency, a book is born. This process has been amazing, and the completion of this book would not have been possible without the following special people in my life, whom I am grateful for.

One of the biggest reasons I am here today is because of my parents, Reeva and Bharat Singh, who have encouraged me and loved me so unconditionally and selflessly. Thank you, Mum and Dad, for being such a tremendous influence and inspiration in my life and for growing me up with the understanding that anything is possible. You have both, been so loving, kind, caring and supportive and have always believed in me. No words could truly express the extent of my gratitude. My dear brother Himal, thank you for all that you have done for me. You have impacted my life and my achievements in so many ways and continue to inspire me with your talents. Thank you for your love, guidance and support, throughout my journey.

Joanne Jasienczyk, you are extremely special to me and have been my pillar of strength since moving to Canada, motivating me continuously and keeping me going. I appreciate you so much and truly grateful for all that you have done for me. Thank you, Joanne.

Gloria Moorhouse, thank you for always listening to me daily, bouncing off ideas, believing and having faith in me and cheering me on with bursts of encouragement. To the Tabor family, Medimax team, Palliotis, thank you for your encouragement and support always. My deep appreciation to my dearest, friends and family, who have encouraged and supported me, in all my endeavours. You have been extraordinary. Thank you.

References

Chapter 1

1. Pascual, L.A. (2018). *A Guide to cognitive fitness*. Harvard Medical School: Harvard Health Publishers. Available at: https://www. harvardhealthonlinelearning.com (Accessed: 8 March 2018).
2. Cortright, B. (2016). *Practical cognitive enhancement: the neurogenesis diet*. Available at: https://www.youtube.com/ watch?v=8qELJTRLJyM (Accessed: 9 April 2017).
3. Amen, D.G. (2015). *Change your brain, change your life*. Available at: https://www.audible.com (Downloaded: 8 June 2017).
4. Dow, M. (2015). *The Brain fog fix*. Available at: https://www. audible.com (Downloaded: 9 May 2017).
5. Kang, J.X., & Gleason E.D. (2013). 'Omega-3 Fatty acids and hippocampal neurogenesis in depression'. *CNS Neurol Disord Drug Targets*, 12(4): pp. 460—5.
6. Kiecolt, G.J.K., Belury, M.A., Andridge, R., Malarkey, W.B., Glaser, R. (2011). 'Omega-3 supplementation lowers inflammation and anxiety in medical students: a randomized controlled trial,' *Brain Behav Immun*, 25(8): pp. 1725-34.
7. Chih-chiang, C., Liu, J.P., Su, K.P. (2008). 'The use of Omega-3 fatty acids in treatment of depression.' *Psychiatric Times*, 25(9): 76-80.

8. Uttara, B., Singh, A.V., Zamboni, P., Mahajan, R.T. (2009). 'Oxidative stress and neurodegenerative diseases: A review of upstream and downstream antioxidant therapeutic options'. *Curr Neuropharmcol*, 7(1): pp. 65-74.

9. Xu, Y., Lin, D., Li, S., Li, G., Shyamala, S.G., Barish, P.A., Vernon, M.M., Pan, J., Ogle, W.O. (2009). 'Curcumin reverses impaired cognition and neuronal plasticity induced by chronic stress.' *Neuropharmacology*, 57(4): pp. 463-71.

10. Shezard, A., Rehman, G., Lee, Y.S. (2013). 'Curcumin in inflammatory diseases.' *Biofactors*, 39(1): pp. 69-77.

11. Hucklenbroich, J., Klein R., Neumaier, B., Fink, G.R., Schroeter, M., & Rueger, M.A. (2014). 'Aromatic-tumerone induces neural stem cell proliferation in vitro and in vivo'. *Stem Cell Research & Therapy*, 5:100.

12. Dias, G.P., Cocks, G., do Nascimento B.M.C., Nardi, A.E., Thuret, S. (2016). 'Resveratrol: A potential hippocampal plasticity enhancer'. *Oxid Med Cell Longevity*: 9651236. doi: 10.1155/2016/9651236. Epub. May 25.

13. Hornsby, A.K., Redhead, Y.T., Rees, D.J., Ratcliff, M.S., Reichenbach, A., Wells, T., Francis, L., Amalden, K., Andrews, Z.B., Davies, J.S. (2016). 'Short-term calorie restriction enhances adult hippocampal neurogenesis and remote fear memory in a Ghsr-dependent manner'. *Psychoneuroendocrinology*, 63: pp. 198-207.

14. Perlmutter, D. (2013). *Grain brain*. Available at: https://www.audible.com. (Downloaded: 9 July 2017).

15. Dow, M. (2018). *Heal your drained brain*. Available at: https://www.audible.com. (Downloaded: 6 February 2018).

16. Harris, D., Adler, C., Warren, J. (2017). *Meditation for fidgety skeptics*. Available at: https://www.audible.com. (Downloaded: 3 Jan 2018).

17. Mirescu, C., Peters, J.D., Noiman, L., & Gould, E. (2006). 'Sleep deprivation inhibits adult neurogenesis in the hippocampus by elevating glucocorticoids'. *PNAS*, 103 (50): pp. 19170-19175. Available at: https://doi.org/10.1073/pnas.0608644103.

18. Leaf, C. (2016). *Think and eat yourself smart*. Available at: https://www.audible.com. (Downloaded: 29 March 2017).
19. Jensen, K. (2016). *Three Brains*. Coquitlam, BC: Mind publishing Inc.
20. Lakhiani, V. (2016). *Code of the extraordinary mind*. Available at: https://www.audible.com. (Downloaded: 4 December 2017).
21. Graham, G.L. (2012). *The powerful impact of food on epigenetics*. Available at: *https://www.youtube.com/watch?v=8X61zvgRKFQ*. (Accessed: 18 June 2017).

Chapter 2

1. Emmons, R.A., & McCullough, M.E. (2012). *The Psychology of Gratitude*. Oxford University Press. DOI:10.1093/acprof:oso/9780195150100.001.0001
2. Emmons, R.A., McCullough, M.E. (2003). 'Counting blessings versus burdens: an experimental investigation of gratitude and subjective well-being in daily life.' *Pers Soc Psychol*, 84(2): pp. 377-89.
3. Hawkins, D.R. (2015). *Letting go: The Pathway of Surrender*. Available at: https://www.audible.com. (Downloaded: 13 March 2017).
4. Dow, M. (2015). *The Brain fog fix*. Available at: https://www.audible.com (Downloaded: 9 May 2017).
5. Dow, M. (2018). *Heal your drained brain*. Available at: https://www.audible.com. (Downloaded: 6 February 2018).
6. Amen, D.G. (2015). *Change your brain, change your life*. Available at: https://www.audible.com (Downloaded: 8 June 2017).
7. Orloff, J. (2009). *Emotional freedom*. Available at: https://www.audible.com (Downloaded: 8 August 2017).
8. Orloff, J. (2009). *Emotional freedom practices*. Available at: https://www.audible.com (Downloaded: 10 September 2017).
9. Lakhiani, V. (2016). *Code of the extraordinary mind*. Available at: https://www.audible.com. (Downloaded: 4 December 2017).

10. Leaf, C. (2016). *Think and eat yourself smart*. Available at: https://www.audible.com. (Downloaded: 29 March 2017).
11. Grace, A. (2018). *This Naked mind*. Available at: https://www.audible.com. (Downloaded: 15 February 2018).
12. Hudson, G. (2018). *Affirmations: Powerful affirmations to empower the subconscious mind to achieve anything*. Available at: https://www.audible.com. (Downloaded: 27 April 2018).

Chapter 3

1. Cornah, D. (2006). *Feeding minds: The impact of food on mental health*. London: Mental health foundation.
2. Selhub, E. (2015). 'Nutritional psychiatry: Your brain on food'. *Harvard Health Publications,* 16 November. Available at: http://www.health.harvard.edu/nutritional - psychiatry - your - brain - on - food - 201511168626
3. Jensen, K. (2016). *Three Brains*. Coquitlam, BC: Mind publishing Inc.
4. Holford, P. (2003). *Optimum nutrition for the mind*. London: Piatkus Books Ltd.
5. Dow, M. (2015). *The Brain fog fix*. Available at: https://www.audible.com (Downloaded: 9 May 2017).
6. Lugavere, M., Grewal, P. (2018). *Genius foods*. Available at: https://www.audible.com. (Downloaded: 10 May 2018).

Chapter 4

1. Selhub, E. (2015). 'Nutritional psychiatry: Your brain on food'. *Harvard Health Publications,* 16 November. Available at: http://www.health.harvard.edu/nutritional - psychiatry - your - brain - on - food - 201511168626

2. Lakhan, S.E., & Viera, K.F. (2008). 'Nutritional therapies for mental disorders.' *Nutrition Journal*, 7:2. Doi: 10.1186/1475-2891-7-2.

3. Akohondzadeh, S., Gerbarg, P.L., Brown, R. P. (2013). 'Nutrients for prevention and treatment of mental health disorders'. *Psychiatr Clin North Am*, 36(1): pp. 25-36.

4. Avena, N.E., Rada, P., Hoebel, B.G. (2008). 'Evidence for sugar addiction: behavioral and neurochemical effects of intermittent, excessive sugar intake.' *Neurosci*, 32(1): pp. 20-39.

5. Mysels, D.J., Sullivan, M.A. (2010). 'The relationship between opioid and sugar intake: review of evidence and clinical applications.' *Journal of Opioid Management*, 6(6): pp. 445-52.

6. Canadian Diabetes Association (2018). *Sugars and sweeteners*. Available at: http://guidelines.diabetes.ca/docs/patient-resources/sugars-and-sweeteners.pdf (Accessed 15 July 2018).

7. Canadian Diabetes Association (2018). *Glycemic index food guide*. Available on: http://guidelines.diabetes.ca/docs/patient-resources/glycemic-index-food-guide.pdf. (Accessed on 15 July 2018).

8. Holford, P. (2003). *Optimum nutrition for the mind*. London: Piatkus Books Ltd.

9. Dow, M. (2018). *Heal your drained brain*. Available at: https://www.audible.com. (Downloaded: 6 February 2018).

10. Pedre, V. (2015). *Happy Gut*. New York: Harper Collins Publishers.

11. Osttman, E., Granfeldt, Y., Persson, L., Bjorck, I. (2005). 'Vinegar supplementation lowers glucose and insulin responses and increases satiety after a bread meal in healthy subjects.' *European Journal of Clinical Nutrition* 59(9): pp. 983-8.

12. Perlmutter, D. (2013). *Grain brain*. Available at: https://www.audible.com. (Downloaded: 9 July 2017).

13. Hadjivassiliou, M. (2002). 'Gluten sensitivity as a neurological illness'. *Journal of Neurology and Neurosurg Psychiatry*. 75(5): pp. 560-3.

14. Jackson, J.R., Eaton, W.W., Cascella, N.G, Fasano, A., Kelly, D.L. (2012). 'Neurologic and psychiatric manifestations of celiac disease and gluten sensitivity.' *Psychiartr Q*, 83(1): pp. 91-102.

15. Canadian Celiac Association and Dietitians of Canada (2018). *Gluten-free eating*. Available at: https://www.celiac.ca/cms/wp-content/uploads/2018/05/Gluten-Free-Eating-PEN. (Accessed 10 June 2018).

16. Bartholomew, A., Monson, N. (2015). *Making sense of vitamins and minerals*. Harvard Medical School: Harvard Health Publishers. Available at: www.health.harvard.edu (Accessed: 19 August 2017).

17. Bottiglieri, T. (1996). 'Folate, vitamin B12, and neuropsychiatric disorders.' *Nutr Rev*, 54(12): pp. 382-90.

18. Coppen, A., Bolander, G.C. (2005). 'Treatment of depression: time to consider folic acid and vitamin B12.' *Journal of Psychopharmacol*, 19(1): pp. 59-65.

19. Bell, I.R., Edman, J.S., Morrow, F.D., Marby, D.W., Mirages, S., Perrone, G., Kayne, H.L., Cole, J.O. (1991). 'B complex vitamin patterns in geriatric and young adult inpatients with major depression.' *Journal Am. Geriatr Soc*, 39(3): pp. 252-7.

20. Eby, G.A., Eby, K.L (2010). 'Magnesium for treatment-resistant depression: a review and hypothesis.' *Med Hypotheses*, 74(4): pp. 649-60.

21. Abdou, A.M., Higashiguchi, S., Horie, K., Kim, M., Hatta, H., Yokogoshi, H. (2006). 'Relaxation and immunity enhancement effects of gamma-aminobutyric acid (GABA) administration in humans.' *Biofactors*, 26(3): pp. 201-8.

22. Grace, A. (2018). *This Naked mind*. Available at: https://www.audible.com. (Downloaded: 15 February 2018).

23. Axe, D (2018). *How does alcohol affect the brain (it's not pretty)*. Available at: https://draxe.com/how-does-alcohol-affect-the-brain/ (Accessed: 20 February 2018).

24. Shi, J., Yu, J., Pohorly, J.E., Kakuda, Y. (2003). 'Polyphenolics in grape seeds-biochemistry and functionality.' *Journal Med Food*, 6(4): pp. 291-9.

Chapter 5

1. O'Mahony, S.M., Clarke, G., Borre, Y.E., Dinan, T.G., Cryan, J.F. (2015). 'Serotonin, tryptophan metabolism and the brain-gut-microbiome axis.' *Behav Brain Res,* 277: pp. 32-48.
2. Foster, J.A., McVey, N.K.A. (2013). 'Gut-brain axis: how the microbiome influences anxiety and depression.' *Trends Neurosci,* 36(5): pp. 305-12.
3. Zhou, L., Foster, J.A (2015). 'Psychobiotics and the gut-brain axis: in pursuit of happiness.' *Neuropsychiar Dis Treat,* 11: pp. 715-723.
4. Wall, R., Cryan, J.F., Ross, R.P., Fitzgerald, G.F., Dinan, T.G., Stanton, C., (2014). 'Bacterial neuroactive compounds produced psychobiotics.' *Adv Exp Med Biol,* 817: pp. 221-39.
5. Jade, K. (2018). *The best probiotics for mood: Psychobiotics may enhance the gut-brain connection.* University Health News. Available at: https://universityhealthnews.com/daily/depression/the-best-probiotics-for-mood-enhancing-the-gut-brain-connection-with-psychobiotics/ (Assessed on: 15 July 2018).
6. Ghodarz, A., Poor, K.Z., Ebrahimi, M.T., Jafari, P., Akbari, H., Taghizaheh, M., Memarzadeh, M.R., Asemi, Z., Esmaillzadeh, A. (2016). 'Clinical and metabolic response to probiotic administration in patients with major depressive disorder: A randomized, double-blind, placebo-controlled trial.' *Nutrition,* 32(3): pp. 315-320.
7. Messaoudi, M., Lalonde, R., Violle, N., Javelot, H., Desor, D., Nejdi, A., Bisson, J.F., Rougeot, C., Pichelin, M., Cazaubiel, M., Cazaubiel, J.M. (2011). 'Assessment of psychotropic-like properties of a probiotic formulation (Lactobacillus helveticus R0052 and Bifidobacterium longum R0175) in rats and human subjects.' *British Journal of Nutrition,* 105(5): pp. 755-64.
8. Kato, K.A., Nishida, K., Takada, M., Suda, K., Kawai, M., Shimizu., Kushiro, A., Hoshi, R., Watanabe, O., Igarashi, T., Miyazaki, K., Kuwano, Y., Rokutan, K. (2016). 'Fermented milk containing Lactobacillus casei strain Shirota prevents the onset of physical symptoms in medical students under academic stress.' *Benef Microbes,* 7(2): pp. 153-6.

9. Liang, S., Wang, T., Hu, X., Luo, J., Li, W., Wu, X., Duan, Y., Jin, F. (2015). 'Administration of Lactobacillus helveticus NS8 improves behavioral, cognitive, and biochemical aberrations caused by chronic restraint stress.' *Neuroscience,* 3(310): pp. 561-77.
10. Dow, M. (2018). *Heal your drained brain.* Available at: https://www.audible.com. (Downloaded: 6 February 2018).
11. Perlmutter, D. (2015). *Brain Maker.* New York: Little, Brown and Company.
12. Pedre, V. (2015). *Happy Gut.* New York: Harper Collins Publishers.
13. Selhub, E.M., Logan, A.C., Bested, A.C. (2014). 'Fermented foods, microbiota, and mental health: ancient practice meets nutritional psychiatry.' *Journal of Physiological Anthropology,* 33:2. Doi: 10.1186/1880-6805-33-2.
14. Campos, M (2017). *Leaky gut: What is it, and what does it mean for you?* Harvard Health Publications, 22 September. Available at: https://www.health.harvard.edu/blog/leaky - gut - what - is - it - and - what - does - it - mean - for - you - 2017092212451.
15. Leaf, C. (2016). *Think and eat yourself smart.* Available at: https://www.audible.com. (Downloaded: 29 March 2017).
16. Maroon, J.C., Bost, J.W. (2006). 'Omega-3 fatty acids (fish oil) as an anti-inflammatory: an alternative to nonsteroidal anti-inflammatory drugs for discogenic pain.' *Surg Neurol,* 65(4): pp. 326-31.
17. Johanna, N. (2016). *Guide to collagen for women.* 21 February. Available at: http://www.nataliejohanna.com/blog/2016/2/collagen - supplements - women.
18. Varani, J., Dame, M.K., Rittie, L., Fligiel, S.E.G., Kang, S., Fisher, G.J., Voorhees, J.J. (2006). 'Decreased collagen production in chronically aged skin.' *Am J Pathol,* 168(6): 1861-1868.

Chapter 6

1. Morris, M.C., Tangney, C.C., Wang, Y., Sacks, F.M., Bennett, M.D., Aggarwal, N.T. (2015). 'MIND diet associated with reduced incidence of Alzheimer's disease.' *Alzheimer's Dementia*, 11(9): 1007-1014.
2. Collins, R., Buckley, S. (2015). *The Mind diet*. South Denver Cardiology Associates. 15 June. Available at: https://www. southdenver.com/wp - content/uploads/2012/09/Mind - Diet-for-web.pdf
3. Morris, M. (2017). *Diet for the mind*. Available at: https://www. audible.com. (Downloaded: 25 December 2017).
4. Lugavere, M., Grewal, P. (2018). *Genius foods*. Available at: https:// www.audible.com. (Downloaded: 10 May 2018).
5. Jensen, K. (2016). *Three Brains*. Coquitlam, BC: Mind publishing Inc.
6. Bayer-Carter, J.L., Green, P.S., Montine, T.J., VanFossen, B., Baker, L.D., Watson, G.S., Bonner, L.M, Callaghan, M., Leverenz, J.B., Walter, B.K., Tsai, E., Plymate, S.R., Postupna, N., Wilkinson, C.W., Zhang, J., Lampe, J., Kahn, S.E., Craft, S. (2011). 'Diet intervention and cerebrospinal fluid biomarker in amnestic mild cognitive impairment.' *Arch Neurol*, 68(6): pp. 743-51.
7. Gyurkovics, M., Kotyuk, E., Katonai, E.R., Horvath, E.Z., Vereczkei, A., Szekely, A. (2016). *Conscious Cognition*, 42: 1-8.
8. Kotler, S. (2014). *Create a work environment that fosters flow*. Harvard Business Review. 6 May. Available at: https://hbr. org/2014/05/create - a - work - environment - that - fosters - flow
9. Bonaiuto, M., Mao, Y., Roberts, S., Psalti, A., Ariccio, S., Cancellieri, U.G., Csikszentmihalyi, M. (2016). 'Optimal experience and personal growth: flow and the consolidation of place identity.' *Front Psychol*, 7:1654. Doi: 10.3389/fpsyg.2016.01654
10. Yoto, A., Motoki, M., Murao, S., Yokogoshi, H. (2012). 'Effects of L-theanine or caffeine intake on changes in blood pressure under physical and psychological stress.' *Journal of Physiological Anthropology*, 31(1):28. Doi: 10.1186/1880-6805-31-28

11. Kimura, K., Ozeki, M., Juneja, L.R, Ohira, H. (2007). 'L-theanine reduces psychological and physiological stress responses.' *Biol Psychol*, 74(1): 39-45.

12. Crook, T., Petrie, W., Wells, C., Massari, D.C. (1992). 'Effects of phosphatidylserine in Alzheimer's disease.' *Psychopharmacol Bull*, 28(1): 61-6.

13. Crook, T., Tinklenberg, J., Yesavage, J., Petrie, W., Nunzi, M.G., Massari, D.C. (1991). 'Effects of phosphatidylserine in age-associated memory impairment.' *Neurology*, 41(5): 644-9.

14. Hirayama, S., Terasawa, K., Rabeler, R., Hirayama, T., Inoue, T., Tatsumi, Y., Purpura, M., Jager, R. (2014). 'The effect of phosphatidylserine administration on memory and symptoms of attention-deficit hyperactivity disorder: a randomized, double blind, placebo-controlled clinical trial.' *Journal of Human Nutr Diet*, 27(2): 284-91.

15. Kim, H.Y., Huang, B.X., Spector, A.A. (2014). 'Phosphatidylserine in the brain: metabolism and function.' *Prog Lipid Res*, 56(1):1-18.

16. Jongkees, B.J., Hommel, B., Kuhn, S., Colzato, L.S. (2015). 'Effect of tyrosine supplementation on clinical and healthy populations under stress or cognitive demands – a review.' *Psychiatr Res*, 70:50-7.

Chapter 7

1. Riebl, S.K., Davy, B.M. (2013). 'The hydration equation: update on water balance and cognitive performance.' *ACSMs Health Fitness Journal*, 17 (6):21-28.

2. Cornah, D. (2006). *Feeding minds: The impact of food on mental health*. London: Mental health foundation.

3. Holford, P., Cass, H. (2001). *Natural highs*. London. Piatkus Books Ltd.

4. Holford, P. (2003). *Optimum nutrition for the mind*. London: Piatkus Books Ltd.

Chapter 8

1. Mayer, E. (2016). *The Mind-Gut Connection: How the hidden conversation within our bodies impacts our mood, our choices and our overall health.* Available at: http://www.audible.com. (Downloaded: 10 October 2017).
2. Vartanian, L.R., Kernan, K.N., Wansink, B. (2016). 'Clutter, chaos and overconsumption: The role of mind-set in stressful and chaotic food environments.' *Environment and Behavior.* Doi: 10.1177/0013916516628178.

Disclaimer

This publication contains the ideas and opinions of the author. It is intended to provide helpful and informative material on the subjects addressed in the publication. It is sold with the understanding that the author and publisher are not engaged in rendering medical, health, or personal professional services in the book. The reader should consult his or her medical, health or other competent professional before adopting any of the suggestions in this book or drawing inferences from it.